Computer-Based Examinations
for Board Certification

Computer-Based Examinations
for Board Certification

Elliott L. Mancall, M.D.
Philip G. Bashook, Ed.D.
J. Lee Dockery, M.D.
Editors

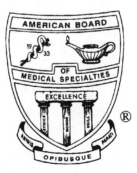

American Board of Medical Specialties®
Evanston, Illinois
1996

Other Books Published by the
American Board of Medical Specialties®

Evaluation of Noncognitive Skills and Clinical Performance, Edited by John S. Lloyd, Ph.D., 1982.

Evaluating the Skills of Medical Specialists, Edited by John S. Lloyd, Ph.D., and Donald G. Langsley, M.D., 1983. (Out of print)

Oral Examinations in Medical Specialty Board Certification, Edited by John S. Lloyd, Ph.D., 1983.

Legal Aspects of Certification and Accreditation, Edited by Donald G. Langsley, M.D., 1983. (Out of print)

Computer Applications in the Evaluation of Physician Competence, Edited by John S. Lloyd, Ph.D., 1984.

The Residency Director's Role in Specialty Certification, Edited by John S. Lloyd, Ph.D., 1985.

Trends in Specialization: Tomorrow's Medicine, Edited by Donald G. Langsley, M.D. and James H. Darragh, M.D., 1985.

Hospital Privileges and Specialty Medicine, Edited by Donald G. Langsley, M.D. and Mona M. Signer, 1986. (Out of print)

How to Evaluate Residents, Edited by John S. Lloyd, Ph.D. and Donald G. Langsley, M.D., 1986.

Recertification for Medical Specialists, Edited by John S. Lloyd, Ph.D. and Donald G. Langsley, M.D., 1987.

How to Select Residents, Edited by Donald G. Langsley, M.D., 1988.

Hospital Privileges and Specialty Medicine, 2nd Edition. Edited by Donald G. Langsley, M.D. and Beauregard Stubblefield, M.B.A., 1992.

Health Policy Issues Affecting Graduate Medical Education, Edited by Donald G. Langsley, M.D., J. Lee Dockery, M.D., and Peyton Weary, M.D., 1992.

The ABMS Handbook on Board Certification and the Americans With Disabilities Act (ADA), Edited by Philip G. Bashook, Ed.D. and J. Lee Dockery, M.D., 1992.

The Ecology of Graduate Medical Education, Edited by Alexander J. Walt, M.B., Ch.B; Philip G. Bashook, Ed.D.; J. Lee Dockery, M.D.; Barbara S. Schneidman, M.D., M.P.H., 1993.

Recertification: New Evaluation Methods and Strategies, Edited by Elliott L. Mancall, M.D., and Philip G. Bashook, Ed.D., 1994.

Assessing Clinical Reasoning: The Oral Examination and Alternative Methods, Edited by Elliott L. Mancall, M.D., and Philip G. Bashook, Ed.D., 1995.

ISBN: 0-934277-22-2

Library of Congress Catalog Card Number: 96-86080

Copyright © 1996 American Board of Medical Specialties®

All rights reserved

Desktop publishing: Gail A. Strejc, American Board of Medical Specialties®

Printed in the United States of America

Contents

v

Preface

Experts on standardized examinations (psychometricians) predict that computer-based examinations are the wave of the future. By the future, the psychometricians mean within the next five years. Many large scale examinations in the United States such as college admissions tests, graduate school entry examinations, and licensure examinations in a number of professions, including some health professions, already have shifted from paper-and-pencil tests to computerized examinations. Among the 24 Member Boards of the American Board of Medical Specialties (ABMS) two boards (the American Boards of Pediatrics and Pathology) offer some of their examinations in a computer-based format. Three more boards (the American Boards of Family Practice, Internal Medicine, and Radiology) are in the research and development stage for converting to computer-based testing.

The shift to realistic simulations on computers, however, has only begun. Experts in computer simulations predict it will be only a few years before clinical performance can be assessed (e.g., procedural skills, clinical reasoning, clinical diagnoses) using case simulations on computers. Experts in "virtual reality environments" (VR), realistic computer simulations, predict VR availability in less than ten years in most academic centers. VR can be used for planning surgery, and for training/evaluating physicians in ways similar to how airline pilots are evaluated. Commercially available examples of VR environments in medicine already exist.

In 54 years of ABMS educational conferences only four have included scientific exhibits with examples of computer-based testing. In 1974, the *Conference on Recertification* used five demonstration exhibits for participants to learn about current assessment technology. Two of the five demonstrations included computer-based "branching-type patient management problems." A summary report on the conference acknowledges the technical feasibility of testing by computer, but stresses the need for further research and development before using computers for board certification. An ABMS conference with computers as the focus was held in 1983, *Computer Applications in the Evaluation of Physician Competence*. The conference included a number of exhibits by organizations using computers in medicine, but few focused upon computer-based assessment. An international joint conference by the ABMS and the Royal College of Physicians and Surgeons of Canada was held in 1988. Demonstrations and exhibits contained six examples of computer-based assessment. The present conference is the fourth and was held in 1996 with 14 scientific exhibitors. All the exhibitors demonstrated some aspect of computer-based testing technology.

These proceedings report on the 1996 ABMS educational conference convened on March 21-22, 1996, at the Westin O'Hare Hotel in Chicago. The conference topic was *Computer-Based Examinations for Board Certification: Today's Opportunities and Tomorrow's Possibilities*. In attendance were more than 250 individuals including some of the leading experts in computer-based testing and medical virtual reality simulations. In contrast to the 1974 and 1983 conferences, by 1996 the conference could draw upon many years of experience in computer-based testing from a variety of organizations. The 1996 conference addressed two questions:

1. Why use computer-based examinations for board certification?
2. Based upon actual experiences with computer-based examinations, how can computers be used to assess knowledge, performance, and judgement as a part of a board certification program?

The invited speakers and exhibitors were selected because they are the most knowledgeable and experienced in using computer-based examinations and computer-based simulations. Many conference registrants provided additional expertise during audience discussions.

The conference welcome was given by **Maurice J. Martin, M.D.**, Immediate Past President of the ABMS. **Elliott L. Mancall, M.D.**, Chairman of the ABMS Committee on Study of Evaluation Procedures (COSEP), served as the conference moderator. Recognizing that some readers of these proceedings may not be familiar with the jargon of computer-based testing, **Philip G. Bashook, Ed.D.**, ABMS Director of Evaluation and Education, prepared a chapter after the conference on basic concepts of computer-based testing (See Introduction).

The keynote address was presented on Thursday evening, March 21, 1996, by **Michael J. Ackerman, Ph.D.**, Assistant Director for High Performance Computing and Communications at the National Library of Medicine, who spoke about *Advances in computer technology for specialty board certification* (See Part 1). Dr. Ackerman provided a multimedia "tour" commenting on older computer simulations (10 years old) through the current computer technology and likely future computer capabilities. During the presentation the technical limits and conceptual advances were described. Following the keynote address, conference participants adjourned to the exhibit hall to visit the scientific exhibits by organizations demonstrating: operational computer-based testing programs; offering expertise in how to convert to computer-based testing; examples of research and development projects for computer-based testing; and hands-on examples of virtual reality simulations in medicine. Conference participants reported the scientific exhibit format stimulated informal dialogue among exhibitors, conference faculty and registrants. Breaks from the plenary sessions throughout the conference were held in the exhibit hall. (See Appendix I for a description of exhibits.)

On Friday, March 22, 1996, the conference continued with a session on the nuts-and-bolts of computer hardware and software for computer-based examinations (See Part 2). **Richard J. Rovinelli, Ph.D.**, Rovinelli Associates and a consultant to the American Board of Family Practice and the American Board of Pathology, used colorful anecdotes to illustrate his recommended list of 18 critical decisions every organization must make in planning to use computer-based examinations. **Gerald A. Rosen, Ed.D.**, Senior Consultant to Sylvan Technology Centers, described the opportunities and limitations of using single testing sites versus multiple testing sites with frequent and even daily test administrations. **Charles B. Johnston, Ph.D.**, Vice President of Sylvan Prometric, provided an overview of the latest developments in technology available at multi-site testing centers and offered advice about how to select testing centers.

The second session on Friday morning addressed the psychometric aspects of computer-based testing (See Part 3). **John J. Norcini, Ph.D.**, Executive Vice President for Evaluation and Research at the American Board of Internal Medicine, described the important psychometric distinctions between computer-based testing and conventional paper-and-pencil testing without once using a Greek letter or equation. Following Dr. Norcini's presentation, **Charles B. Friedman, Ph.D.**, Professor at the University of North Carolina (and co-author, Stephen M. Downs, M.D.), discussed recent research on how to score complex clinical case simulations using a "decision-theoretic approach." "Decision-theoretic approaches" are based on Bayes' theorem of conditional probabilities. The next session provided three examples of successful conversions to computer-based testing (See Part 4). **Anthony R. Zara, Ph.D.**, Director of Testing for the National Council of State Boards of Nursing, described the Council's seven-year experience from initial decisions to current use of computer-based testing to examine 200,000 nurses annually for state licensure. **William H. Hartmann, M.D.**, Executive Vice President of the American Board of Pathology, discussed the board's experiences from the perspective of the board staff and trustees in designing a computer-testing center to assess pathologists. **Fred G. Smith, M.D.**, Vice President of the American

Board of Pediatrics, offered lessons learned and diplomates' reactions to the board's "take-home" computer-based recertification program for board certified pediatricians.

The conference then focused upon lessons learned about computer-based simulations (See Part 5). **Donald E. Melnick, M.D.**, Senior Vice President at the National Board of Medical Examiners (NBME), described the important conceptual and technical advances and lessons learned during a nearly 30-year odyssey by the NBME to introduce computer-based clinical case simulations into physician licensure examinations. **Colonel Richard M. Satava, M.D.** (and **Lieutenant Commander Shaun B. Jones, M.D.** as co-author), Program Manager, Advanced BioMedical Technologies, Advanced Research Projects Agency (ARPA), United States Department of Defense, offered a multimedia presentation on virtual reality (VR) environments in medicine. The last session in the conference was a presentation by **Roger C. Kershaw**, Vice President for Technologies at the Educational Testing Service, in which he described what is currently available in computer-based testing formats and what is likely for the future (See Part 6). Concluding remarks by **William H. Hartmann, M.D.** and **Elliott L. Mancall, M.D.** offered suggestions for continuing the stimulating discussions as an outcome of the conference (also in Part 6). The book also contains appendices and author and subject indices. Appendix I contains a list of conference participants and Appendix II contains a comprehensive bibliography on computer-based examinations.

Elliott L. Mancall, M.D.
Philip G. Bashook, Ed.D.
J. Lee Dockery, M.D.
Editors

Acknowledgments

These conference proceedings were prepared to memorialize the papers and discussions presented at the March 21-22, 1996 conference on *Computer-based Examinations and Board Certification: Today's Opportunities and Tomorrow's Possibilities.* Conceived by the Committee on Study of Evaluation Procedures (COSEP) of the American Board of Medical Specialties (ABMS), the conference was planned by a subcommittee of COSEP: Fred G. Smith, M.D., Chair (American Board of Pediatrics), Elliott L. Mancall, M.D. (Chair, COSEP), William H. Hartmann, M.D. (American Board of Pathology), Gerald P. Whelan, M.D. (American Board of Emergency Medicine), and Philip G. Bashook, Ed.D. (ABMS staff). The conference's success is due in large measure to the thoughtful and dedicated work of the planning subcommittee members, the excellent presentations by the 12 conference faculty, the superb exhibits by 13 organizations who are experienced, knowledgeable, and helpful in computer-based testing, and virtual reality simulation, including five Member Boards of ABMS, and the insightful comments and discussions from the 250 conference participants.

Thanks and appreciation are conveyed to a number of people: to Maurice J. Martin, M.D. (ABMS Immediate Past President), whose leadership and commitment to board certification are manifest in his continued strong support of these conferences; to the ABMS staff who were extraordinarily helpful as always; to J. Lee Dockery, M.D., Executive Vice President of ABMS, without whom none of this could have happened; and to Philip G. Bashook, Ed.D., Director of Evaluation and Education of ABMS and the staff person for COSEP. In that role he has made important contributions in both conceptualizing and implementing the conference program.

I would also like to thank the members of COSEP, all of whom have shared in conceiving the conference: George E. Cruft, M.D., Joel A. DeLisa, M.D., Stewart B. Dunsker, M.D., Francis P. Hughes, Ph.D., Edward A. Krull, M.D., Mary Ann Reinhart, Ph.D., and Fred G. Smith, M.D.

A special thanks is due the ABMS staff who produced these proceedings: Gail Strejc for her work in type-setting the manuscript for desk-top publishing, Alexis Rodgers for guiding the publication process, and Marci Burr, Bobbye Higdon, Evalyn Moore, and Kathleen Hoinacki for their secretarial efforts.

Elliott L. Mancall, M.D.
Chairman, ABMS Committee on Study of Evaluation Procedures
Co-Editor

INTRODUCTION

Concepts of Computer-Based Testing
for the Novice

Introduction

Concepts of Computer-Based Testing for the Novice

Philip G. Bashook, Ed.D.
American Board of Medical Specialties

Advances in computer technology have brought the use of computers into the forefront of testing and assessment of physicians and other professionals. It is common today to observe directors and trustees for certifying boards debating the merits and obstacles in converting current paper-and-pencil tests to computer formats. In fact, many of the discussions and even some of the more impassioned debates can be explained by differences in interpreting exactly what is meant by computer-based testing.

Having participated in the conference, and having overheard casual conversations where at least one of the participants spoke in "technospeak," it became apparent to me that it would be helpful to have a layman's explanation of the arcane concepts and language of computer-based testing. This chapter is in response to those observations. It was prepared after the conference and is designed to provide the novice in computer-based testing ("CBT") a beginning vocabulary for conversing with more sophisticated colleagues.

Explanations are grouped into categories to correspond with these proceedings, and when searching for reference articles. Appendix II contains a bibliography to begin the search. Every effort has been made to use straightforward language in translating the computer-testing jargon in this chapter; apologies are extended where "technospeak" encroaches on the explanations. Of course, any translation of technical terms cannot entirely convey their exact meaning or subtle nuances. It is hoped, however, that these efforts will be successful in launching those interested on a safe journey through "CBT."

3

The reader will note that the terms "computer-based testing" and "computer-based examinations" are used as if they are synonymous. Although many might dismiss this as a non-distinction, others would argue strongly that "testing" means standardized tests in the multiple-choice format while "examination" implies a variety of different testing formats. No position is taken here in this debate, but the issue is aired because the terms do have subtly different technical meanings. The terms "test item" and "test question" are used here interchangeably as well.

Test Formats

To begin at the beginning is to plan an examination program. Computers may not be uppermost in the minds of a test committee while they develop a test, but decisions about computer-based testing must begin with the test plan or test blueprint.

The *test blueprint* defines the scope and depth of content to be tested. For each concept or fact, the test blueprint states whether candidates will be tested for ability to reason as a professional, remember the fact or concept, or interpret the findings as presented in the test question (usually a clinical case example). The blueprint also specifies the number of test questions to be included for each content area.

The test blueprint is an essential template for deciding which computer-based test format to use. Conforming to a test blueprint is achieved more easily by mixing different test formats in a computer-based test than with a paper-and-pencil test.

Multiple-Choice Questions (MCQs) -- Many experts in psychometrics advocate using the MCQ format to measure recall of knowledge, interpretation of data, and, when designed appropriately, problem solving ability. Each multiple-choice question in typical standardized tests begins with a brief paragraph containing the essential information and a question (called the "stem"). A candidate responds to the question by selecting one of four or five choices (called "distractors."). One distractor is keyed as the correct answer. The candidate records a choice on a computer-coded answer sheet. The test is scored by computer programs designed to scan each coded answer sheet and produce test statistics and a score, or scores, for each candidate. There are many variations on this paper-and-pencil MCQ format. A most helpful book on MCQs is by Thomas Haladyna.[1]

Multiple-choice questions were one of the first test formats to be widely incorporated into computer-based testing. Some computer enhancements of MCQs use video clips or sound effects as part of the question "stem." Large typefaces are easily created on computer screens for assisting candidates with visual impairments. Creative variations occur routinely for computer-based MCQs.

Some of the common terms used in describing computer-based test formats are:

Linear tests -- Linear tests are essentially the computerized version of paper-and-pencil MCQs. Test questions in the MCQ format are presented on the video screen one at a time in a linear fashion. The questions may include pictures, and even audio with video displays. The sequence of questions may vary for each candidate, as with different versions of a standardized test, but the number of questions and the content covered is based upon the test blueprint. Candidates answer each question by touching a key on the computer keyboard. Computer-based "linear tests" can be programmed to allow candidates to mark questions for later review. In essence a linear test is administered on the computer in nearly the same way as using test booklets and computer-coded answer sheets.

Computer adaptive tests -- Computer adaptive tests (CAT) present candidates with a sequence of test questions (nearly always in MCQ format) carefully selected by question difficulty to pinpoint the candidate's level of ability. The CAT computer algorithm is programmed to select questions individualized for each candidate, shifting back and forth between easy and hard questions until a good estimate of the candidate's ability can be established. Some candidates can have a short test while others may require many test questions before their ability has been estimated. In CAT most candidates receive about one-third to one-half the questions given in a linear test; the testing time can be reduced accordingly. CAT requires a larger pool of test questions compared to linear tests, on average 1000 questions. It is an evolving test format that is becoming more widely accepted in the general testing community.

Constructed-response items -- The multiple-choice question and other test formats using lists of options can provide a hint to some candidates who may not know the correct response. By asking candidates to construct a response to a question rather than choose from a set of distractors, this "cueing effect" can be eliminated. This test format is most helpful when assessing problem solving ability or ability to interpret data, but candidates usually take longer to complete the constructed-response items compared to MCQs. Some examples of computer-based constructed response questions are: answering a question by giving a short sentence answer or even a brief paragraph using the computer's word processing capability; performing mathematical calculations by using the calculator on the computer and scoring the answer directly from the calculator display; drawing on the screen to mark the limits of a lesion on an x-ray or patient image, or to identify the location of a surgical incision, or where to position a prosthesis. Computers make possible a unique testing opportunity by allowing candidates to "drag" an image (picture, words, equation, or any defined "object") across the screen and position it near another image or object. In computer-based testing these test items are called "drag and drop" questions.

Computer Simulations -- Simulations are computer representations of actual situations the candidates are expected to encounter. They are used to measure the candidate's ability to solve a clinical problem or demonstrate clinical reasoning skills. A "high fidelity simulation" would represent a real situation as closely as feasible with the available technology. Typically, simulations start as clinical cases either in text, pictures, or video clips, to introduce the "opening scene" and present the candidate with the clinical problem. In some simulations the candidate navigates through decisions about diagnosing the case using only word lists. In other simulations candidates can navigate by typing an answer, moving ahead a simulated clock, or using the computer mouse to retrieve a specific laboratory report, a nurse's note, or x-ray display. In Part 5 of these proceedings, Dr. Donald Melnick describes the history of such a computer case-based simulation developed by the National Board of Medical Examiners. In Appendix II refer to references #18, #76, #78, #82, #84 for more on simulations.

Virtual reality simulations (VR) -- Virtual reality simulations are computer-generated environments in which people can interact with the environment and with other people. VR test questions combine the benefits of constructed response questions and of simulations, adding the realism of actual clinical situations. VR has the potential to measure procedural skills, clinical judgment, and problem solving ability. Candidates are presented a very realistic clinical situation (very high fidelity but simulated), and interact in the virtual environment using the same medical devices they would use in practice. The devices are attached to the computer and use manikins in place of live patients. The term for these computer devices is "haptic interfaces." They have sensors linked to the computer to give candidates the feel of real movement. Images in the VR environment change to match the candidate's actions. In some commercially available VR environments the candidate holds a real scalpel or tissue probe, a gastroscope or a bronchoscope and interacts as if the patient were "real." Precise measurements can be obtained and scored for the candidate's positioning of the device, insertion or probing, and tissue repair or removal. Adding realistic complications to VR simulations is possible as well as simulating the evolving nature of a disease or patient condition to test how well a candidate responds. The better designed simulations resemble "real time" patient management and provide a means for standardized performance measurements not possible with real patients. Part 5 contains a more detailed description of VR by Drs. Satava and Jones.

The **Test item bank** is the term for computer storage of test questions. Test item banks store not only each question but detailed information about the question. Typical information linked to each question includes: key words defining the content covered by the question; the candidate's ability level to be measured; a record of which tests contained the question; every version and revision of the question (revisions to both the stem and distractors); a record of the question author(s); statistics on the question difficulty, reliability, and other measurements; and notations on the pictures or images, x-rays, or videos used with the question. Computer programs are written to retrieve questions with all the attached data and to select questions for constructing a new test according to a test blueprint.

Test Administration by Computer

If you have a driver's license you may have taken a computer-administered driving test at a motor vehicle department. Most driver testing centers use a central computer connected to terminals. The candidate sits at a table facing the terminal, follows the instructions on the screen, and answers a series of multiple-choice questions by touching a key on the keyboard. This is a *test administered by computer.* The transmission between the computer and the terminals occurs concurrently for everyone in the room, even though each person may not be answering the same questions. Offering tests simultaneously at multiple sites around the country involves basically the same process.

Examinations for professional certification usually use personal computers (PCs) instead of terminals connected to a central computer. Unlike PCs, terminals have little computer memory and no hard disk drives for data storage. The PCs, with significant amounts of memory and hard disk drives, are placed in cubicles or stations. Partitions between stations separate candidates to enhance privacy, reduce noise, and lessen opportunities for cheating. Sometimes the PCs are free-standing with the test on a diskette or each PC's hard drive. In other centers the PCs function as terminals connected by cables to the central computer at that testing center in a *local area network, or LAN.* In LANs a central PC controls PCs at each station. When the candidate finishes, a file is transmitted electronically back to the central computer for analysis. In free-standing PCs the diskettes with the candidate's responses are removed by the proctor or the candidate's test data is copied off the PC's hard disk drive and analyzed.

Data Transmission

Most multiple-choice questions on computer use only text and do not need to transmit data at very high speeds. When pictures, sound or video-images are included the computer hardware (computers, monitors, and cables) needs to be fast and efficient. High resolution images (i.e., quality images), video clips and sound necessitate rapid transmission of large amounts of data. With video clips the video monitor must be refreshed rapidly or the picture will flicker or appear fuzzy. Some terms for computer speed and central processing units (CPU) chips are "megabytes," (i.e., "processor speed in megahertz"), CPU chips like the Intel® 486SX® or 486DX4®, "Pentium®" or "Pentium Plus®". The language for cables connecting PCs includes "band width," "twisted pair 10 Base–T wiring," or "T1 cables." Sometimes this "technospeak" sounds more like the name of a new rock band, but be forewarned, Part 2 contains papers using these terms. Very secure data transmission is technically feasible in a LAN (local area network) within a single location or large networks linking computers worldwide using the *Internet.* Connecting computers brings to the fore issues of security. More information about computer security can be found in Appendix II

(See references #70 to #75; reference #75 is an *Internet* address with information on security).

This introductory journey through the computer-based testing language was written for those who want a beginning vocabulary. Once you delve into the remaining chapters it is hoped you do not find the jargon overbearing; there is much to be learned from the computer testing pioneers who contributed to these proceedings.

Reference

1. Haladyna, TM. *Developing and Validating Multiple-Choice Test Items.* Hillsdale, New Jersey: L. Erlbaum Associates. 1994.

ADVANCES IN COMPUTER TECHNOLOGY FOR BOARD CERTIFICATION

PART

1

BOOK RECEIPT

PERMANENT LOAN ☑

PERSONAL GRANT ☐

NAME _____Cuevas_____

PRICE _____$48.95_____

INVOICE #_____prepaid_____

VENDOR _____ABMS_____

P.O. # _____L32964_____

FUND #_____1000-4-1100-510_____

AUTHOR _____

TITLE_____Computer-Based Examinations
for Board Certification_____

date rec'd. _____9-11-96_____

Advances in Computer Technology for Specialty Board Certification

Michael J. Ackerman, Ph.D.
National Library of Medicine

In thinking about the use of computers for board certification examinations, I realized that talking to this audience is like preaching to the church choir. Most of you have extensive experience in the use of computers for competency testing. You know its history and you know its benefits. For those that do not have that background, it is very simple: It is desirable in competency testing to test the candidate in the same situation and under the same conditions in which the candidate would be expected to practice. One way to do this would be in the clinic. One could find patients with the appropriate conditions, bring them to the clinic, and have the candidate work them through. Another way would be to use a computer to simulate the clinical environment and the patient. The problems encountered in developing computer simulations for medical training and testing will no doubt be discussed by other speakers at this conference. I decided, therefore, to look at this issue from the point of view of technology:

- What technology has been tried in the past?
- What technology is currently available?
- What technology might be used in the future?

One of the issues that is always discussed when one talks about technology is the interface between the human and the computer. In the testing situation, the question may be stated as, "How much do I have to know about the interface in order for it not to interfere with the testing process?" Or, "Am I being tested on my knowledge of the subject matter or am I being tested on my computer skills?" For this discussion assume that an interface can be built which is transparent, which will absolutely not interfere with the testing process. Why can I make such an assumption? Because such an interface has already been developed in the

11

airline industry, for the post office, and in welding. Welders are tested and certified using simulators! They do not have problems with the interface interfering with testing. Neither do airline pilots. The problem of developing a transparent interface for medical training and testing can be solved by answering two questions:

(1) How much money are we willing to spend to solve the problem?
(2) How long will it take the entertainment industry to solve the problem for us?

Either way, it is solved. The problem is currently unsolved because we, all of us, have not raised the economic stakes high enough in medical training and testing. People do not realize the liability of not testing doctors in the same way that airline pilots are tested. Somehow, the lives that are entrusted to airline pilots are of greater value than the lives that are entrusted to doctors. The airline industry has the economic support to be able to develop the needed interface and we in medicine do not.

I will, therefore, make the assumption that the problem of a transparent interface is an economic or a timing problem, not a technical one. It will be solved. If nothing else, it will be solved by the entertainment industry and we will benefit from it. This is the traditional way that technology is developed for computer-based instruction and computer-based testing. Some of my colleagues might argue the point, but I will use the terms computer-based instruction and computer-based testing interchangeably because, from a technological point of view, they are one and the same.

When I was the Chief of the Educational Technology Branch of the National Library of Medicine (NLM), the common wisdom was that computer-based instruction would rapidly find its place in medical training because the National Board of Medical Examiners (NBME) would be testing competency through the use of its computer-based examination. We felt that medical students, rightfully or wrongfully, would say, "Since you are testing me by computer, I am entitled to learn by computer. You should teach me in the mode in which I will eventually be tested." So, computer-based testing was linked to computer-based instruction because they are based on the same kind of technology. The NBME computer-based examination had not been instituted, computer-based training went largely unused, and the common underlying technology went undeveloped.

The biggest impediment to using computer technology for either teaching or testing in medicine is the limitation of rapid transmission of pictures. It is easy to create a computer-based examination composed solely of text. That is the equivalent of the current paper-and-pencil examination. Using a computer for text could offer ten or fifteen choices instead of the paper-based four or five choices. The computer can score fifteen choices as easily as four choices. But, technically they are basically equivalent multiple-choice tests.

When a candidate examines a patient, the patient does not present the case by saying, "Doctor, I have a pain in my left biceps muscle with an occasional episode in my triceps muscle. Therefore, I have:

A. Tennis elbow
B. Sore arm
C. . . . ."

That is not real. In reality the patient says "Doctor, it hurts here!" There are unlimited choices and no prompts. Paper-based examinations do not allow such unlimited possibilities. On the other hand, computer-based examinations can display a picture and ask a question, and candidates can choose an answer by pointing to the proper structure on the picture or by typing the answer in common language. The responses are captured by the computer and may be scored immediately. The score can then be used to suggest the next appropriate question.

This kind of open environment always raises the problem of geographic differences in what should be considered as the proper answer. When I was a little bit younger and was working in biomedical engineering, people would ask "What do you really do?" and I would say "Neurophysiology." I could tell where a physician was trained based upon how he or she applied the EEG (electroencephalogram) electrodes to a patient. It is surprising how specific training location influences clinical technique. Despite the differences in technique, recordings of patients' EEGs were equally successful. But, in the EEG laboratory people would individually and unequivocally state that the technique they used to apply EEG electrodes was the only technique that would result in proper EEG recordings. For some the technique was as simple as wiping off the skin with an alcohol pad and pasting on the electrodes. Others would literally use sandpaper until the skin almost bled. Yet the quality of the recorded EEG signals was the same. Depending on the training of the grader, the comments might read "You inflicted too much skin trauma," or "You did not do enough skin cleaning." But the quality of the recorded signals was the same. Thus, there are geographic differences in clinical style. We must be aware of them because the openness of the computer-based examination will heighten their effect.

The biggest impediment to using computer technology for either teaching or testing in medicine is the lack of ability to transmit pictures rapidly. The main channel to the human brain is the eye. It is the channel with the largest band width. Ninety percent of the information we encounter comes through our eyes. I believe that much of what a physician bases a diagnosis on is not necessarily what the patient tells him or her, but what is seen. Although the written interpretation of images is often part of the differential diagnostic process, actually looking through the microscope, looking at the x-ray, looking at the patient, or looking at other visual results is usually much more instructive. There is a story in the annals of computerized diagnosis about a research group studying artificial intelligence that was developing a diagnostic program. The proper tests were run, the diagnostic information was entered into the computer, and the computer made a diagnosis. The patient was then presented to a physician with 40 years of experience who made a diagnosis. The physician was correct and the computer was wrong. The computer logic was checked and there were no errors. How could this be! The physician agreed that the logic was correct, but not in this case. Why not in this case? The physician explained that when he came into the room and saw the way the patient was lying on the bed he knew the diagnosis. This is an element of art, and it is channeled through the eyes.

A technology is needed that would allow us to see, that will allow us to participate. Heart sounds, chest sounds and bowel sounds are part of the diagnostic process. At NLM, when discussing technology for medical diagnosis, Dr. Donald A. B. Lindberg (Director of NLM) reminds everyone that there is nothing like "thumping on the tummy to diagnose a problem." So technology needs to allow us to see, to hear, and to feel.

Using the NLM archives, let us look at the progress in computer technology beginning about ten years ago. Then let us move forward and see how this technology progressed, and finally look forward and make an educated guess about what technology will be available in the not-too-distant future.

Figure 1

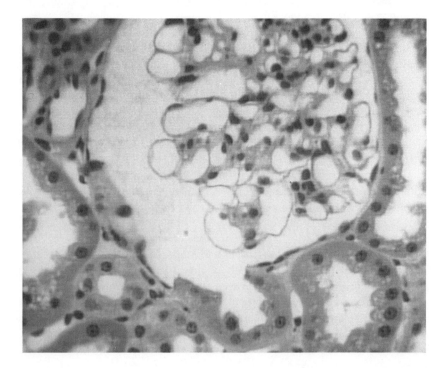

Some will remember the National Library of Medicine's Human Light Microscopy project. It was based on a videodisc that was produced by NLM. Histological images were captured on video tape and put on a videodisc. A computer interface made it possible to look at an image of a single slide to determine what it was (Figure 1).

Push a key on the computer's keyboard and labels would appear on the image (Figure 2).

Figure 2

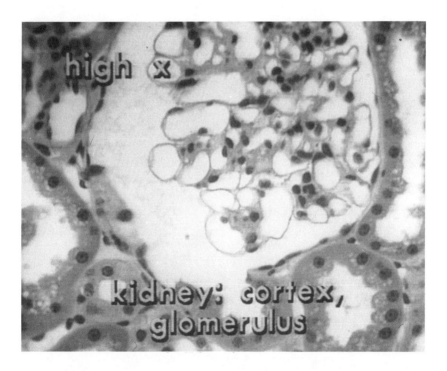

It could be used for instruction or for self-testing. The pictures were presented by way of the videodisc.

Eight to ten years ago, when this program was produced, high resolution images could not be stored or presented by the computer. At that time the state-of-the-art in affordable computer color displays was called EGA color. It had limited resolution and it was capable of displaying only sixteen colors—not nearly enough to display realistic histological images. Computers were used to control the videodisc players; the images were provided from videodiscs. It was the state-of-the-art. It was considered to be remarkable.

Many people consider computer use to be too difficult to master. Computer phobia is not a new condition, so the manufacturers of videodisc players developed a bar code system to control the players. The medical community developed videodisc-based educational materials using the bar code system. A book contained the bar codes and labeled sketches of their associated images.

Figure 3

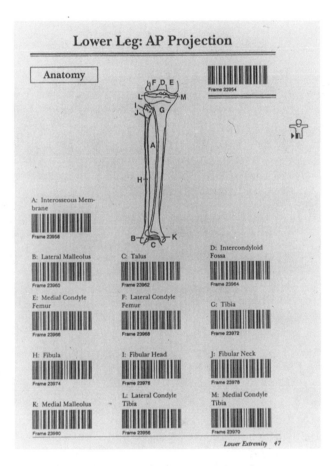

The bar code wand was traced over the bar code and the full color labeled image contained on the videodisc was displayed on the screen. The system also can be used in a testing situation. For example, a student displays the image of an unlabeled sketch controlled by a bar code.

Figure 4

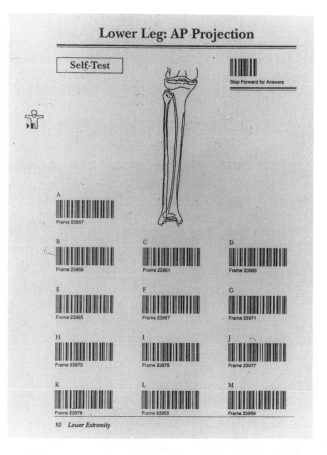

The image is displayed from the videodisc without labels. The paradigm is similar to the light microscopy example but this example does not use the computer.

NLM's Knee Anatomy program used a videodisc, computer, and touch screen. It was designed for the self-study of cross-sectional knee anatomy. First, labeled cross-sectional images are shown.

Figure 5

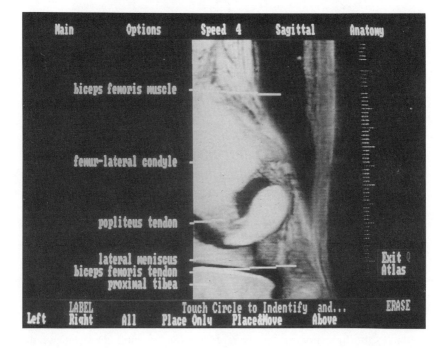

Then the same images are displayed with circles around each of the parts. To name each of the parts one touches the appropriate circle. When a circle is touched the label reappears.

Figure 6

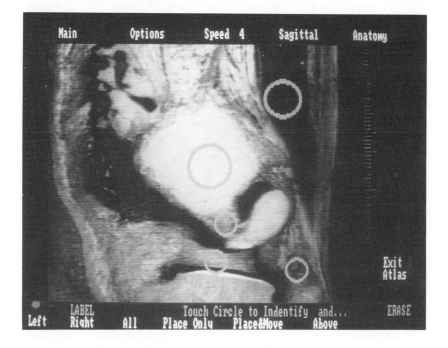

Finally, unmarked images are given and students are asked to touch a particular anatomical part.

Figure 7

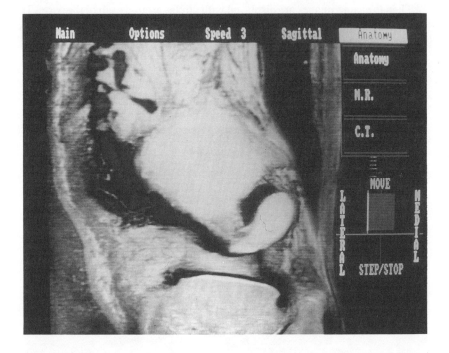

The touch sensitive screen allows the computer to know where the student is pointing and, therefore, whether or not it is the correct answer. These pictures are displayed from a videodisc but the labels and circles are provided by the computer in an overlay mode. Overlay technology was very expensive at the time but was required in order to be able to display images of reasonable quality.

The National Board of Medical Examiner's Computer-Based Examination (CBX) was also based on videodisc technology. The computer presents a patient: "A 65-year-old man with a history of . . ." and so on. The program contains a clock. The case is being timed, which provides some realistic pressure. Time is moving right along and you have to move along with it. The student asks for the patient's history and a written summary appears on the screen. Based on the history, tests, drugs, or whatever else that might be appropriate can be ordered. It is not multiple choice. There are thousands of possibilities available. The computer reacts to each of them in the appropriate length of time. The student can wait for the results or speed up the simulation by letting the computer know that he or she wants to advance the clock to look at the test results. The machine will move the clock forward. As time progresses the student can be "paged" and given the nursing notes stating the patient is having trouble. It is now up to the student to respond. Do something about it now, or wait until the tests come back?

CBX tries to engage the student in a realistic simulation. But it is not realistic enough. It does not give a true sense of reality because most interaction with this simulation is through text. It is not the experience a student or physician would have if he or she were really present with a live patient. It requires the student's imagination to get involved in the experience. Considering that it is an examination, I am confident students can be very motivated. The technology is a bit primitive, however, compared to the technology available today.

It is true a patient's chest film could be seen on the TV monitor, but the TV monitor does not provide enough resolution to properly display a full chest film, so students had to choose which part of the film to display and move from part to part.

Figure 8

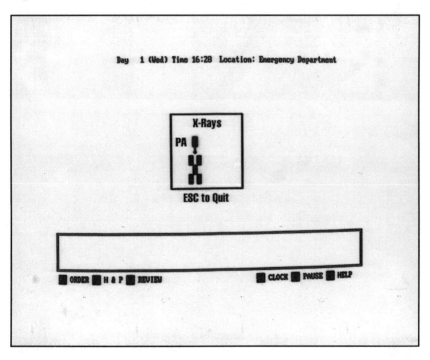

Likewise, if an electrocardiogram was ordered, the choice was to see the 12-lead cardiogram or the rhythm strips.

Figure 9

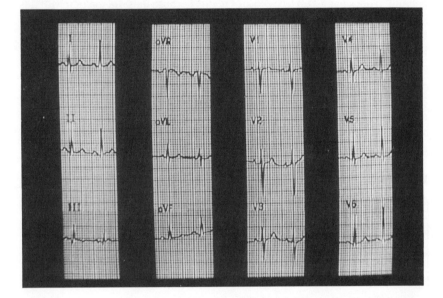

Figure 10

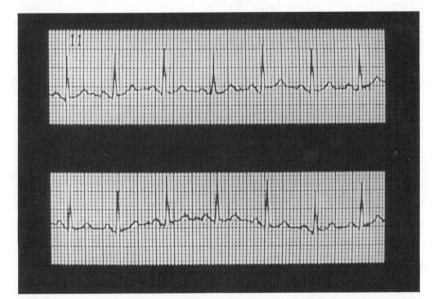

The idea is to work up and to manage the patient. Actions are recorded and form the basis for scoring performance.

Other simulations were written which prompted more dynamic student interaction. These simulations used a computer and touch screen to control motion. One of the simulations in the DXTER simulation series is a "Shot Gun Wound to the Abdomen" that takes place in an emergency room. This shotgun wound example was shown in the TV series *St. Elsewhere.* An intern on rotation in the emergency room was not allowed to progress until he passed an examination consisting largely of this simulation. It has been used for testing, but was originally designed as a teaching tool.

Another example was "Mediquiz," a simulation designed by the military to teach and test hospital corpsmen.

The technology to provide real-time realistic simulation is called "virtual reality." It can be used to help students feel that they are part of the reality, that the patient is really in front of them. In order to make a patient seem real, pictures of the patient must be displayed in rapid succession. This is a technological challenge. The chart (Figure 11) shows how long it would take to transmit a single x-ray film, 2,000 points by 2,000 points by 4,000 shades of gray, at different communication rates. Several years ago, when this chart was put together, the most common rate was 2,400 baud. At that rate it would take six hours to send the X-ray film. Obviously this was not going to work for virtual reality. But even if we go to a T1 line (special high-speed data line), today's institutional standard at the equivalent of 1,500,000 baud, it still takes 32 seconds to move this kind of an image.

Figure 11

Transmission Times for a Digital Chest Film
(2,000 points by 2,000 points by 4,000 shades of grey)

Line Type	Bits Per Second	Transmission Time
2400 baud	2,400	6 hours
9600 baud	9,600	1.5 hours
56 kilobaud	56,000	15 minutes
T-1	1,500,000	32 seconds
Ethernet	10,000,000	5 seconds
T-3	45,000,000	1.25 seconds

Many may know of my involvement in the Visual Human Project™. An x-ray film image contains many fewer data points than a single Visible Human anatomical image. A single Visible Human image would take even longer to transmit. So in order to move an image in less time, it either has to move faster or it must be made smaller. Reducing the number of data points while preserving the image is a process called "compression." Compression is the mathematical process of eliminating the redundancy from the picture. You start with a picture, compress it (i.e., eliminate the visual redundancy) so it is made up of fewer data points, and it can be transmitted in less time. Before it is displayed at the TV receiver, it is expanded back to its original size. But, since the compression process eliminated what was mathematically considered as visually redundant, the result is a loss of resolution.

Figure 12

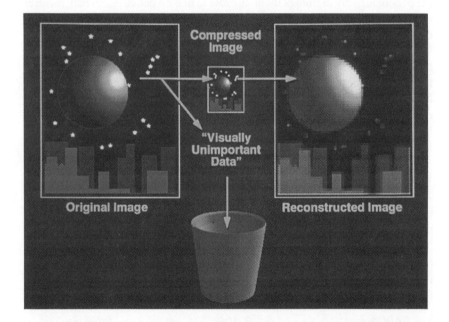

In Figure 12, stars are still there but they are not quite as clear; the globe is not as round as it used to be; and the landscape again has changed. In many cases, that which is considered as visually redundant by some, may actually make the difference between making and not making a diagnosis for others. So, we have to be very careful in using compression technology. Medicine must go beyond what the entertainment industry will use. Their definition of what is visually redundant for entertainment is radically different, and the visual loss that can be tolerated for games, may not be acceptable in medicine.

Here are some examples of compression. Suppose a figure is 512 dots wide by 480 dots high. One way to compress an image is to sample it with fewer dots. In this case it could be 64 dots wide by 60 dots high. The compressed image requires 64 times less space than the original image. It takes 1/64 the time to transmit it. The image is not as clear because it has less resolution. This type of reduced clarity is known as "pixilation." For someone who is using the image to identify a person, it is not likely to be a problem; but, try making a dermatological diagnosis and the compressed image is probably useless.

The FAX machine rapidly transmits an image through a different type of compression. The grey tones in a facsimile are first converted to either black or white; there is no grey. The person is recognizable but does the picture have any diagnostic value? What if the picture was an x-ray, just black and white and no grey? As the grey tones are put back you can begin to see the shading. But as these grey tones return, the picture in the digital world takes more storage space and more time to transmit. A picture with 256 grey tones requires eight times the storage space as the same image rendered in just black and white.

There are two modes of storing the digital data needed by computer-based testing programs. The data can be stored locally or it can be stored somewhere on a network. If it is stored on a network, one faces the problem of obtaining image data fast enough to display it as a true motion image; this is the technical challenge of compression.

Pictures received over the Internet and World Wide Web can be very complicated, but Web transmission is not difficult provided one is patient. The testing environment requires rapid transmission times. If images cannot be provided very rapidly, it becomes an annoyance and interferes with the testing environment by distracting the student. Therefore, the current trend is to store the needed data locally. Sometimes remarkable things can be done locally on small machines: An ophthalmic simulator for example, was programmed by High Techsplanations for use on a Macintosh® computer.

Another approach is not to use a general purpose computer as the simulator, but to build a special purpose simulator very much like the cockpit simulator used to train and evaluate pilots. Instead of using an available state-of-the-art Macintosh® or PC, suppose we built a special purpose simulator out of available off-the-shelf equipment which could simulate the actual touch and feel of the patient. A practical example is the virtual endoscopy simulator built by Axion.

In this simulation the motion is smooth while in the ophthalmic simulation the moving images have a staccato-like flavor. That staccato-like flavor is generally acceptable and is believed not to interfere with the student really feeling immersed in the simulation. The endoscopy simulator was developed about five years ago and uses analog videodisc technology. It is now being redeveloped using digital video technology on CD-ROM. It can now be substituted transparently for the videodisc.

A state-of-the-art celiac plexus simulator was recently developed by the University of Colorado Medical Center in Denver based on data from the Visible

Human Project.™ The simulation allows the student not only to see, but also to feel the tissues as a needle is pressed through the skin and toward the celiac plexus. It is current state-of-the-art. It can be done. It takes two powerful computers and some equipment that is not quite off the shelf. I have tried it and it actually works.

The last example is not available today, but is likely for tomorrow. The example has a student at the University of California, San Diego, working through a test project in managing a patient. The student speaks to the computer and the computer responds using natural speech. The computer has instant access to all the needed data bases including image sets. The human-machine interaction is as easy and natural as studying with a colleague.

The ability to program this complicated simulation is well into the future and many technologies must be developed first before this simulation becomes reality. Initially, the necessary clinical and epidemiological databases must exist. Further development in voice recognition technology is needed to allow the student to be understood by the computer. But these technologies are coming; their seeds already exist.

During this conference and beyond, keep your horizons high. Do not say it is impossible. The last example is possible, it will just take some time. I encourage you to remain aware of the state-of-the-art of the technological tools needed to accomplish your tasks, and be ready to use them, because it is only a matter of time before they become practical.

HARDWARE AND SOFTWARE

Balancing Price, Versatility
and Obsolescence

Richard J. Rovinelli, Ph.D.
Rovinelli Associates

For a number of years I have been involved with several organizations in the design, development and implementation of computer-based testing programs. In the past two years I have had the opportunity to work with two medical specialty boards in their computer-based testing programs, the American Board of Family Practice and the American Board of Pathology. What has become apparent to me is that even though many of these organizations have different goals and objectives for their testing programs, they share concerns about hardware and software, and their selection and purchase.

This presentation starts with the premise that the medical specialty boards are at an historical watershed with regard to computer-based testing. The watershed is very similar to what the boards faced in the late 1940s and early 1950s when they decided to shift from essay examinations to the multiple-choice or "objective" format. It is my belief that all of the medical specialty boards will, in a relatively short period of time, utilize computer-based testing programs in one form or another for certification or recertification. If the form of utilization happens to be a high stakes or pass/fail decision, then they will need to make a series of decisions:

1. Either develop the software or create test centers with their staffing and computer equipment.

2. Utilize the services of vendors such as those presenting at this conference—high quality people with high quality products.

3. Some combination of the two, developing software and utilizing those services.

29

Regardless of the strategies used, specialty boards will have to make a series of decisions and conduct an evaluation. Today I plan to share some of the information accumulated while working with these organizations, and describe what I call the *ouch factor*, some of the mistakes made in the decision processes by not looking carefully enough at the full ramifications of possible decisions before taking action. As background, I am a psychometrician by formal training, a computer programmer and analyst by technical training, but neither a hardware expert nor a communications technology expert.

An analogy to what boards face is the relationship between the primary care physician and the specialist. The primary care physician needs to know the limits of their knowledge and when they need to go to specialists to get that information. I have prepared a list of tasks, by no means exhaustive and additions are welcome, that you need to "know" and to "do" to implement a computer-based testing program.

Common questions I will answer are: What is the process? What do I have to go through? What are the kinds of things with which I have to deal? What do I have to address in order to implement these programs successfully? This presentation provides:

1. A list of tasks useful for deciding about purchasing hardware and software.

2. A working definition of hardware and software obsolescence.

3. Recommended ways to reduce the impact of hardware on software obsolescence.

4. Examples of balancing price with performance. If you want the performance, you have to pay the price. In some instances you have no choice but to get the "highest end" equipment available in order to implement a program.

1. Develop a list of goals.

The first task in planning computer-based testing programs is to develop a list of goals, i.e., to define the reasons for wanting to use computer-based testing. Is it because you went to an ABMS conference and somebody said that is the direction to go? Or, are there fundamental goals to be achieved? It is important to state the goals clearly: whether to replace a written examination, develop better reporting mechanisms, administer examinations multiple times during the year (which is very difficult and costly with paper-and-pencil testing), design new mechanisms for testing clinical reasoning, or expand the way information is presented to physicians (e.g., videos, sound, images). With a list of goals for implementing the testing program, identify those that are essential, that you will not back off from, and those that are on the wish list and would be nice to achieve but are not essential. Start with the goals for the decision process.

2. Create a budget.

I often hear, "How can I create a budget when I really don't know what I'm going to be doing?" Well, work backwards. For example, how many people are tested in a written examination format, and the oral examination, for boards who use this test format? How much money is spent on the examination at this time? Can the board afford to increase the testing budget by 25 percent (i.e., raise candidates' fees 25 percent)? If the answer is *No*, then the budget for the computer-based test should be established at the level of current testing expenditures. If the objective is to decrease costs associated with the examination program, then the starting budget becomes the current budget minus a given amount of money. These budgets are a point of reference from which you can start making decisions. Establishing a budget is very important in setting appropriate implementation targets.

Included in budget estimates are such items as: the initial start-up costs, the developmental costs, costs for creating centers (if these are contemplated), contract or service costs, and ongoing maintenance costs. If vendors are used, costs will increase slightly each year and contract costs should be budgeted anticipating an incremental charge. Another, often hidden, expense is the administrative cost for the examination.

3. Establish the number of sites or geographic locations required for effective implementation.

Currently, there may be 50 sites or 100 sites around the country where the examination is given. These multi-site administrations set a level of expectation for candidates. More centers mean that candidates do not have to travel too far because increased travel means increased expense for the candidates. If the plan for computer-based testing assumes one center, then the board has made a very important decision. Decide up front whether or not the board can take the "political hit" associated with going from 50 testing centers to one testing center, for example, and balance the "political hit" with the cost implications.

4. Determine the number of years the initial equipment and hardware must last in order to recoup start-up costs and sustain the testing program.

This step concerns deciding how much money it will take to begin and whether candidate fees or other income can be used to recoup the capital investment. Moving into computer-based testing requires a substantial investment. Even if vendors are utilized in some way, there are initial costs. What are those costs? How will the expenses be amortized? These questions lead in turn to further questions, such as: When do you have to begin replacement of equipment and software? How long will the equipment remain current, or the software serve its purpose?

5. Describe in detail the type and features of the testing program which are to be implemented.

Return to the goals and ask, why computer-based testing? What actually will be done? Will there be multiple-choice questions in the computer-based test and is that the primary reason for using computers? Will there be video, sound or still images? What will be the quality of those images? Will the images and video be an integral part of the examinations? Will there be "drag and drop" questions? What about allowing candidates to manipulate questions? Will there be clinical simulations with "real time" interactions?

6. Set the number of test questions in each examination because this determines the amount of testing time required.

Will the testing be a morning session or an afternoon session? Will there be two sessions a day? These decisions have implications in terms of number of sites. How many people will be tested at the sites? With a morning session and an afternoon session, each station can be used twice a day (i.e., two candidates per day). All day testing sessions means one candidate for one station per day. Answering these questions begins the process of creating a checklist for decisions about selecting software and hardware.

7. Determine the software development tool that will be utilized to implement the testing system.

Why is this important? As a rhetorical question, how many walked around the exhibits in the conference and asked what computer language or operating system was used? What system is used? These are very important issues, especially in terms of hardware obsolescence. A good example is the effect Microsoft Windows 95® has had on hardware decisions. Systems with 8 megabytes RAM (random access memory) have difficulty effectively running that operating system. Assume that the software development team expects to use some testing software package that requires 8 Megs of memory and runs on Windows 95®, but the machines available are only 486 Intel® chip machines or slower with only 4 Megs of memory. Obviously, there will be added hardware costs for an upgrade. For an optimum system, what mix of software tools and hardware will be required?

In today's environment information is collected from physicians in an electronic format. That information has to be stored in some form of semipermanent computer program structure, typically organized as a database. There are many different databases available; one is called "client server architect." The American Board of Family Practice's computer-based testing program uses Microsoft's Sequel Server.® This form of software has some significant advantages for the manipulation of data, the storage of data, and the collection of data. It also has significant hardware requirements. At the end of this discussion I will give specific examples and their implications for balancing software selection and hardware requirements.

8. Determine the operating system under which the testing system will be delivered.

Will the operating system be Windows®? Will it be 16-bit Windows® environment (Versions 3.1 or 3.11)? If it is, there will be a major change in a year or so. Clearly, the replacement will not be a 16-bit environment; whether it will be Windows 95®, OS/2® or Windows NT®, (all 32-bit systems), is not clear, but all these environments require significant changes in software from a 16-bit environment. Will Apple computers still be around? They have phenomenal systems, great presentation, great graphics, but will this computer platform exist in ten years?

In making these decisions the board takes on an unknown business partner. Any time one chooses an operating system or hardware, a partner is added. That company is in business to make money. Their decisions will be based, not on *your* needs or requirements, but on *their* needs and requirements. Be aware of the implications of making those kinds of judgments.

9. The work station is very important.

Decisions here concern the appearance of the work station used by the candidate. As I mentioned, I'm not a hardware expert. I have no expectation that the specialty boards employ the type of people that can answer some of these questions. The key point is to understand that there are a series of risks and the implications that flow from hardware decisions. Hardware expertise is needed as part of the planning team, and can be obtained externally through consultation. Work stations can have a significant impact on costs simply by understanding the goals and objectives and the kinds of test items to be displayed. Hardware has its own language, "CD-ROMs", "RISC" systems, "RAM", "SIMMS" slots. It is not necessary to cover each of these today, except to simply say that each one of them can have an impact on what you do.

As a specific example, consider the computer "bus type." This term refers to the speed at which the computer operates internally to move data back and forth. Now the ISA, "industry standards architecture," happens to move data at ten megabytes per second. The PCI (data bus) happens to move it at 100+ megabytes per second. Assume the examinations will use many graphic images. Graphic images take many bytes to transmit. A piece of hardware or a work station that is ISA-based can be bought at a great price, $1,500, while a PCI-based computer might cost $2,900. There is a saving of $1,400 by purchasing ISA work stations. But, now there are major problems in using graphic images because the ISA computers would be too slow. It is important to understand these hardware factors; they are crucial in decision making.

10. Determine the level of fault tolerance in service and down time.

With a paper-and-pencil test, some of the disasters during test administration are hurricanes and tornadoes, or electrical system failure for short periods of time. Over the years, the American Board of Family Practice has had some of these. When the power went out for a period of time in the testing room, we simply waited for it to start again. Maintenance people are called, they make repairs and the testing process continues with proctors keeping the candidates and the testing under control. If a computer server stops working, there are double ramifications for computer-based testing. Quite frankly, there will be fewer test sites as compared to paper-and-pencil tests, with more physicians traveling long distances. It will mean their travel costs will go up, and they might need a hotel room, at least for overnight. If possible, of course, the candidate will want to take the test on one day and leave with no overnight hotel stay. If the computer server or the software, or some hardware, fails, the board cannot just tell the candidates to stay over in the hotel an extra night until the computer is repaired. What kind of redundancies are built into the computer system to protect against such disasters? Here is an example in preparation for the conference exhibit. Two pieces of equipment were brought from Kentucky for the conference exhibits. One computer had programs duplicated on the drive and one part of the hard drive went down. Fortunately, there was a duplicate and it was loaded. If there was no redundancy yesterday, it would have meant serious trouble and no conference exhibit today.

What should be said to a candidate who has been on the system for three hours and the computer malfunctions, losing their test data? "Don't worry, we'll start you off this afternoon." From a psychometric point of view there are serious implications when this happens. Data back up is essential. A number of technologies are available—"RAID technology," and "system fault tolerance," among them. Selecting a software operating system, LAN (local area network) server software and the hardware support will become very important decisions.

11. Determine the local area network (LAN) which will be utilized.

There are a series of choices in local area networks (LAN). Probably the biggest players will eventually be Microsoft NT® and Novell Netware®. Either is a very positive choice. Each has advantages and disadvantages. Understand what those advantages and disadvantages are and what the consequences are of choosing one or the other. Notice, when going to an outside vendor for a quote, that there are still checklist points to review. Ask for information to be confident that the system actually does what it claims. Make sure the testing center is adequate to meet testing needs, not simply the presentation of one test a year, but storage of information, protection of candidate security, and ongoing holding of information.

12. Determine the communication access methods.

Communication access issues are rather esoteric, but important to appreciate. The issue is data transmission between the server and the work station. For example, the American Board of Pathology had a choice last year in putting together the test center. They had a choice and a trade-off. At the time Hewlett

Packard announced a 100 "VG Anycan" **adaptor** that transferred data between the server and work stations at more than 100 megabytes a second, or use Ethernet to transfer data at 10 megabytes a second. Hub switching communication equipment which allows transfer to each of the work stations at 10 megabytes does not require the additional cost for 100 megabyte adapters. Graphics transfer at this slower rate was more than adequate. The decision saved $200 per work station; and with 50-60 work stations, the savings are substantial. This example illustrates why currently available faster technology was not necessary.

13. Determine the LAN topology.

A decision about LAN topology is most important with test centers that have been pre-wired. Assume the board has a testing program and expects to use a commercial testing center with pre-wired work stations. What kind of wire is used in the center between server and work stations? Is it shielded, is it unprotected, does it cross over electrical conduits? How far are the stations from the server? Depending on the type of wire, the distance from the server can create problems in quality of transmission. It is not adequate to just visit a test center and observe them demonstrate two or three work stations in operation. Of course, the stations will run smoothly. Have the center "fire up" all the work stations, and have them demonstrate data transmission to the farthest station. Such a demonstration will help you to appreciate the limits of the LAN, whether it is a vendor or the board's own test center.

14. Determine what "Servers" to use.

The discussion started off with the work stations. My recommendation is to separate the purchase of work stations from buying a server. Most hardware vendors like to package these together; it gives them an opportunity to be flexible in estimating the cost of the hardware and it improves their negotiating strategy. The server really is the guts of the operation. Spend more on the server for two reasons. First, there will be multiple work stations. Every dollar spent on the work stations is multiplied by the number of work stations. Extra expenditures for the server are limited to one or two servers depending on the needs for redundancy and fault tolerance. Second, you should obtain the highest end servers as possible; put as much power in this equipment as you can, both in terms of processing speed and memory. Take advantage of the unique aspects of the operating system. For example, if Novell is used, keep in mind that Novell does a phenomenal job of caching information, storing information in memory and using it. Therefore, you want much more memory. There are significant advantages to looking carefully at system requirements of operating systems.

There are available excellent magazines with advice on the types of work stations and servers. Figure 1 contains a list of journals and magazines that should be in the board office even if the board is not technically oriented or dealer oriented. The magazines cover communications, hardware, software and graphics issues with excellent reviews. For example, a recent issue of *PC Magazine* reviews servers and offers a detailed recommendation with the reasons why. The expertise does not need to be in-house if it can be found elsewhere.

Figure 1

Informative Technical Magazines

Hardware	**Software**
BYTE	BYTE
PC Magazine	PC Magazine
Datamation	Datamation
Office Technology	Application Development Trends
PC World	PC World
LAN Times	LAN Times
Computer Technology Review	Software Development
PC Week	PC Week
	Network Computing
	Network World
	Windows NT® Magazine
	Global Knowledge Network Digest

Multimedia	**Communications**
PC Graphics & Video	Communications of ACM
New Media	Interactivity
3D Design	Communications Systems Design
Computer Graphics World	Enterprise Systems Journal
Digital Video Magazine	Presentations
Multimedia Systems	Communications Week
Imaging Magazine	
AV Video	

---

15. Obtain estimates for each of the components that have to be purchased, including installation and maintenance.

At this point there should be a list of all hardware requirements; wiring requirements have been completed; work station configuration and requirements are set; and the server requirements specified. It is time to get bids, multiple bids on the whole process. This is where the iterative nature of checklists comes into play. When the estimates come back, arrange them in terms of quality—highest to lowest. Go back to the initial budget estimate. How close are these bids to the budget estimate? In the first round it is probable that the budget estimate will be lower than the bids. It is time to return to your goals and objectives for becoming computer-based. Where can there be cuts? For example, was an extra $1,200 added to the work stations because it was expected video would be used but will video be needed now or later, say in two years? If not now, take it off the wish list for work stations. How is that done? Perhaps by reducing from four megabytes to two megabytes of video memory (VRAM) — on the video board. In essence, go back and change the hardware configuration to make it match the budget requirements without compromising the essential goals of the project. But keep in mind which goals are essential.

Where cuts are no longer reasonable, the budget must be reviewed. One option is to raise money to pay for the new system. If that option is not reasonable, it will be necessary to re-evaluate the whole conversion initiative.

16. Obsolescence.

Obsolescence paralyzes all who do not replace their own personal computers on a regular basis. Everyone with a computer has gone through this cycle. Some define obsolescence as: *the availability of software or hardware which provides better performance for a comparable price than existing hardware or software.* Frankly, the day equipment is purchased it is obsolete, by that definition. Every single day there are announcements of new equipment and software. This approach to obsolescence, however, is not the key issue. Here is a case in point:

In 1983 and 1984 my group developed for a pharmaceutical firm a computer testing program with two purposes. The first was to pretest sales people to make sure they had done their homework assignments, and the second was to simulate sales procedures as part of the training session. It was written in interpretative *Basic* language on the initial PC. Five years later I was amazed when I went back to the same pharmaceutical firm as a consultant. The program was still being used. I was embarrassed, having written the code initially, at how long it took the sales representatives to answer the questions. But, to them, this computer-based test was not obsolete. For anybody else in the country, a program written in interpretative "Basic" using these old PCs was an obsolete system. Nobody would put it in that form today. A more reasonable definition of obsolescence is therefore a situation in which,

Existing software or hardware can no longer be utilized to meet the goals and objectives of the testing program.

When making plans, consider the period of time that hardware and software will be useful. For me, the second definition is more reasonable for planning and implementing computer-based testing programs.

There are a number of possible causes of obsolescence:

A. *The organizational goals and objectives for computer-based testing programs are changed or require additional features.* With more experience in computer-based testing, the board's expertise will increase in terms of what can and cannot be done. If the board staff are advanced psychometrically, they will be advanced from a technical point of view and may decide to change the testing program requirements. That decision can introduce obsolescence.

B. *The operating system software has been upgraded but it will no longer support the testing software, the performance is unacceptable, or a new operating system will not run on existing hardware.* This change can be related to the initial decision about choosing an operating system. Remember the partner is a commercial company. Once an operating system is chosen, the company who makes that operating system and those who sell it are your partners. If it is a DOS-based system, it will become more difficult as time goes on to find computers to run it, even though Microsoft, for example, with Windows® 95 and Windows® 3.1, includes DOS availability to run computer code. Eventually a decision will have to be made when the software performance level becomes too denigrated with an older operating system.

C. *The network system software has been upgraded.* Windows NT® can change with newer versions. For example, a work station using a 4.1 version of Windows NT® changes the entire look of the test presentation. The software is completely different. Candidates will need to go through further training to learn to use it. Are disks sent to candidates for practice that have one look on the work station but now a different look on the diskettes? This discrepancy can introduce obsolescence into software and hardware for the work stations.

D. *The existing hardware can no longer be maintained at a reasonable price, or availability of replacement parts is a problem.* This is a typical scenario with computers. Keeping software or hardware over a period of time eventually forces change because the hardware maintenance costs increase and should be anticipated.

These four possibilities of obsolescence exist regardless of how well planned the conversion process and how distant in time the projections for obsolescence.

17. **How to minimize the risk of obsolescence while balancing price and performance?**

A. During any developmental process it is essential that the software development team use the latest tools and versions of the operating system. Make sure the team stays with the software update cycle. Staying with the latest development cycle does two things: it increases team productivity and guarantees that when software has been designed it will be current, thus expanding the projected time for software use before obsolescence.

B. Programming models evolve for any given software developmental effort. The team should use a developmental paradigm which minimizes the task of changing and enhancing the software. The programming team and the developmental team will need a strategy. Are they always working on the basis of a programming paradigm that will allow modifications to the system, replacing certain components rather than rewriting the whole system? It is not cost effective to make total revisions, and it is very important in terms of the developmental cycle of products to use modular programming.

C. Whenever possible, use software development tools that cross over different computer platforms (i.e., DOS®, Windows®, Mac®). In beginning a developmental effort, make sure that the software development tools will run on multiple platforms. This approach builds in some protection and also allows creating mechanisms for handling information changes. For example, Microsoft C++® has a cross platform application in the Mac® (Apple) environment through PowerPoint®. But, Delphi® is problematic because Delphi® is Windows® based. The choice is very important in the developmental effort.

D. Monitor carefully current modifications in the operating systems planned for the testing program. For example, Windows® has had a whole series of releases: alpha, beta, and regular upgrades. Be sure to keep up with those operating system cycles.

E. Hardware should only be purchased after the software has been developed. This is crucial in planning. Making the hardware selection and purchase decision after the software has been developed provides the opportunity for performance simulation. Performance simulation is field testing to assess how well the software performs on different hardware configurations. There are firms that specialize in performance simulations and will provide estimated costs. These companies can target a configuration and actually simulate implementations on work stations. After reviewing the simulation data, revisit the work station and server requirements; then begin to select and purchase hardware.

F. Separate the purchase of work stations and LAN servers. Work stations and LAN servers have different goals and requirements. Ask for separate bids and get the best deal in both separately to maximize the opportunity for hardware selection. Use established criteria to select work stations. Earlier I spoke about having equipment criteria and how those criteria must match the essential goals of the program. Now apply those criteria in selecting work stations. Do the same with regard to selecting the LAN server.

18. **Examples of balancing price and performance.**

To conclude, I have some specific examples of balancing price and performance and also of paying the price to get the performance. A recent example from the American Board of Family Practice is germane. In preparing for this conference, a decision was made to save time and put the work product on a single system. Using a 133 megahertz Pentium® processor with 96 megabytes of memory, Microsoft's Sequel Server® was added to a work station as the client/server environment. The board's server uses parallel processing (i.e., multiple concurrent processing). The algorithm to generate simulated patient cases dynamically generates patients and takes three or four minutes even on a parallel processor system. The patient generation took 20-plus minutes in the single processor work station. This is clearly too long for a demonstration. If the system was initially designed for a single processor, it would have forced a re-look at the developmental work to decide if it needed parallel processing. Current performance simulation projections suggest it will need four processors (two additional) to reduce the patient generation process to just seconds. Clearly, computer processing speed is very important, but we will have to pay the price.

The American Board of Pathology (ABPath) provides an example of a computer-based testing program balancing price and performance with respect to obsolescence. The initial vendor bids in March, 1995, specified an Intel 486 DX4® processor at 66 megahertz. The next generation computer chip up from the 486 system is the Intel Pentium®. At the time, each 486 cost $2,300-$2,400, a good price. Pentiums at the time, were rated at 90 megahertz and sold for $3,000 a work station. The difference would be $600 per work station for 46 work stations. It does not take a mathematical genius to say there is a significant amount of money involved. The board decided not to buy the 486 DX4 system because it was the end of the line for that computer architecture. The Pentium® chip was brand new and would improve.

By spending the $600 extra per work station the ABPath bought themselves a three or four year extension on obsolescence for the work stations. The recent announcement of upgrades on the Pentium® processor from 90 to 133 megahertz, at a couple of hundred dollars each, clearly shows the importance of the purchase decision. But, the upgrade to Pentium® added further expenses to the hardware budget.

Another example linked to this one involves not selecting the most advanced technology. William H. Hartmann, M.D. (Executive Director of the American Board of Pathology) looked at the quality of the images to be displayed at work stations. Two video RAM boards were considered; one costing $400 had 4 Megabytes of video RAM (VRAM) and would give true color, millions of colors. The other was a video card with 2 megabyte VRAM which would only give 16,000 colors on it, but at about half the price. In reviewing the images from the perspective of the pathologist and a candidate taking the test, no differences could be discerned between image quality (16,000 colors versus millions of colors). Clearly, there were differences, but no impact on quality was discerned. The board, therefore, decided to purchase the 2 megabyte VRAM board, thus saving a couple of hundred dollars per board for 46 work stations; this mitigated some of the expense for the higher quality Pentium-based work stations.

With these examples of very practical trade-offs in price and performance, I wish you well in selecting the appropriate hardware and software.

Single Sites, Multi-Sites
and Multi-Day Availability

Gerald A. Rosen, Ed.D.
Sylvan Learning Systems

Computers have been used to administer examinations since the 1970s. However, it is only in the last several years that examinations for purposes of certification have begun to shift in large numbers from paper-and-pencil to computer administration. Computerized testing is having a profound influence on all phases of testing programs by affecting everything from what can be measured efficiently and economically to the ways tests are developed and how they are administered. This paper will briefly review some of the choices to be made in operating a computer-based testing program and some of the consequences of those choices.

Computerized test administration can be performed in a manner very similar to the way paper-and-pencil examinations are administered. Space is secured for use on a single day, usually several times per year, or according to some other part-time schedule. The testing venue may be classrooms in a school or a permanent site. Equipment may be shipped for use on the test day or days and returned afterwards, or may be kept in storage at or near the test site and set up for use on test days. Test administration personnel may be the same individuals who supervise paper-and-pencil administrations, provided they are knowledgeable about the basics of computer usage. Another method of delivering tests via computer is for the organization sponsoring the examination(s) to build its own computerized testing system and one or more test delivery sites. Finally, computerized test administration can also take place at established commercial testing centers staffed by personnel specifically trained for the purpose. A critical feature of this type of computerized testing is that there is a specialized entity, the computerized testing services agency, that has direct control over the staff and sites, makes them available on a five or six day a week

41

basis, and schedules testing appointments for examinees. At any given time at a commercial computerized testing center, one can see examinations from several different testing programs being administered simultaneously to examinees seated at individual, partitioned workstations. Thus, a computerized credentialing examination can be administered at one site or many. It may be made available on one or several days per year, during one or several testing periods or windows of opportunity per year, or on demand throughout the year.

The variables of test sites, one versus many, and test availability, single-day or on demand, can have an impact on examinee convenience, examinee costs, test development costs, organizational costs, organizational control, and security. We will explore these issues in the context of computer-based testing (CBT). Individuals interested in using these issues as a basis for comparisons between computer-based testing and paper-and-pencil testing are referred to *Certification and Licensure Testing: A Comprehensive Resource* to be published later this spring by The National Organization for Competency Assurance.

Examinee Convenience

There is no doubt that the more frequently examinations are available and the more sites at which they are administered, the more convenient it is for examinees. This is true of examinations offered in any form—oral, practical, paper-and-pencil, or computerized. However, not every examination requires hundreds of sites or testing on demand. As the number and geographical dispersion of examinees increase, the need for additional test sites also rises. For examinations with more critical consequences for examinees, increased availability, up to testing on demand, becomes more important. For some certification examinations, two to four test dates or testing windows per year may be sufficient. For other certification examinations and many licensure examinations, testing on demand can have very positive consequences. Examinees passing their test can go to work sooner, work force shortages may be alleviated faster, and temporary licensure can be discontinued. Ending temporary licensure is particularly important because it can carry the possibility of admitting to practice, if only briefly, individuals who may ultimately prove to be unqualified.

For busy professionals, the ability to test on demand on a computer may mean not having to interrupt office hours, hospital rounds, and board meetings in order to sit for an examination.

Examinee Costs

In general, as the number of test sites increases and as test availability increases, candidate costs decrease. It should be noted that examinee costs can include travel, subsistence, lodging, and time lost from work. More test sites means fewer examinees will have to travel to other cities or states, travel costs will be lower and, for some examinees, virtually eliminated. Lodging and subsistence costs similarly will be reduced. For many examinees the most important benefit of increased sites and test availability may be that it will not be necessary to disrupt their usual work schedule. This may be a convenience issue, but it can also be a significant cost issue as well, since the income lost from missed appointments may not be recoverable.

Test Development Costs

Increasing the number of testing sites need not have any effect on test development costs. If examinations continue to be administered on the same number of days each year as they were prior to the increase, the same test development schedule that was in use prior to the increase in test sites may suffice. In other words, if fixed test forms were used, the same number of fixed forms may be all that is required as the number of test sites increases. If an on-line test generation model was being used, then the same item development schedule may serve as well for the increased test sites.

Nonetheless, the effect of increased test availability will be to increase test development costs for most testing programs. The reason for this is the need to minimize threats to examination security that can result from communication between examinees who have been tested and those who are scheduled to test on future dates. There are a number of ways to improve test security: one is to increase the number of test forms in use at any given time for those programs employing fixed forms. Another possibility is to convert from the use of fixed forms to one of the on-line test generation models. Programs using an on-line test generation model can increase the number of items in their item banks so that test generation algorithms select from larger groups of items and, thereby, produce examinations with less item overlap. All the methods involve greater test development efforts, and the additional efforts translate into higher test development costs. On the other hand, some certification programs report that when test sites and availability are increased, participation (i.e., the number of examinees seeking certification) also increases. Thus, the higher test development costs may be at least partially offset by increased revenues received from more candidates.

Administrative Costs

There may or may not be any increase in administrative costs due solely to increasing the number of test sites. If a commercial computer-based testing vendor is delivering the examinations, the entire domestic network of sites is typically included in the test administration fee. If an organization has been operating its own site, moving to a commercial vendor may be more expensive, but on the other hand it may no longer be necessary for the organization to continue to offer tests at its own site. Finally, if an organization operating its own site decides to build out additional sites, there will be very significant additional capital expenditures involved, and additional operational costs for running the sites. This is why it is rare for organizations to consider for long the notion of owning and operating their own testing network. By using a commercial vendor, capital and operational costs are, in effect, shared with the vendor's other clients.

Increasing test availability, like increasing test sites, may or may not affect administrative costs. In this case, however, if costs change they are likely to decrease. If examinations that were offered once or twice a year are administered during one or two testing periods per year there is likely to be little effect on administrative costs. There will be no change in application deadlines and processing schedules. In short, the office staff will continue to work as they always have. If, however, examinations are made available on demand, there may no longer be any need for application deadlines, or at the very least there may only be a need for several rolling deadlines. This change can have the effect of leveling the peaks and valleys of the work loads that are often associated with programs that administer their examinations on yearly or semi-annual cycles. For testing programs with thousands of examinees, a relatively even spread of the processing burden over the full year may mean that fewer permanent and/or temporary staff are required to get the necessary work completed.

Organizational Control

If the highest possible levels of direct control are important to an organization sponsoring a credentialing examination, then that organization ought to consider testing at as few locations as possible and on as few days as possible. This statement stems from the principle that the less there is to control, the more effective the attempts at control will be. Similarly, any organization that requires control at the highest possible level should also administer examinations only at its own test site. By using a commercial computer-based testing vendor, a significant amount of control must necessarily be relinquished to the vendor. It is only the rare testing program, however, that has any great need for such control. Most organizations find it relatively easy to establish a partnership with a computerized test administration vendor and to develop procedures that achieve the organization's testing goals in ways that are quite acceptable. The best course of action may be for organizations that have a very high need for control to do their own test development and their own test administration at their own site.

Security

We have already examined the issue of threats to security posed by communication between examinees. Other security issues include identification and admission of examinees, monitoring of the testing process, and transmission of examinations and/or item banks and examinee performance data to and from test sites. The effect of increased test sites and test availability on examinee identification and admission and monitoring of the testing process is minimal. The only difference is that these functions will be performed in more locations and/or on more days. These functions may be performed in the same ways they were before the changes, or there may be a need for enhanced procedures. For example, some commercial vendors can photograph and thumbprint examinees and videotape testing sessions to provide additional confidence in the integrity of the test administration process.

Data transmission to and from testing centers and data storage at sites are highly technical issues. Clearly, if there is any vulnerability in the transmission process, the threats to security will increase as the number of test sites increase. Increasing the availability of examinations will have a similar effect whether examinations are stored on site in file servers or transmitted to testing centers when examinees schedule their appointments. In either case, there will be longer time periods during which data are vulnerable. However, various data transmission and encryption schemes have been developed to reduce this vulnerability. It appears that in over 16 years of computerized testing by commercial vendors, there has not been a single case of unauthorized data capture either during transmissions or from testing center sites.

Recommendations

In my opinion, the guiding principle for the administration of certification programs is that sponsoring organizations should make the process as easy as possible for the examinees in as many ways as possible, unless there is a very good reason not to. That means examinations should be readily available in as many locations as feasible. Too often, limitations are placed on the number of test sites or availability of examinations because of, for example, the possibility of security problems that have an extremely small likelihood of occurrence. Furthermore, increasing examination availability does not necessarily mean that programs must undergo the expense of developing huge item banks or converting to adaptive testing. The majority of credentialing programs are small enough that simply increasing the number of test forms and administering them in scrambled item order will provide more than the minimum necessary protection from security threats due to communication among examinees. This is not to say that organizations should not adopt adaptive testing if they can afford it and if they feel that the additional expenditures are worth it. The point is that it is not an absolute necessity for many programs. There are many ways to administer examinations acceptably via computer. For the majority of testing programs, it is not necessary to sacrifice examinee interests to do the job well.

Discussion

Robert Greenes, M.D. (Brigham & Women's Hospital, and American Board of Radiology): I noticed that no one mentioned the "I" word or the "W" word—Internet and Worldwide Web. These are factors that are changing how we can build multi-media software and deliver it. There are certainly issues of security, but those are solvable with encryption and password protection. I wonder how that affects some of the decisions that people have made. I notice that none of the exhibits, including our own from the American Board of Radiology, is currently based on the Internet, but there is really no reason that I can see why all the things we have seen cannot be done that way. I wonder if the speakers could comment.

Gerald A. Rosen, Ed.D. (Sylvan Technolgy Centers): Being responsible for some of the technology developments, we, at Sylvan, have taken a look at the Internet and keep looking at it. I think it requires evaluation. I was concerned about some of the security issues, too. A big concern to me, as one with the responsibility to run a global testing network, is for me to have a vendor that I can go to when the communication system does not work. With the Internet it is hard to know who I could approach when it fails. My experience so far has been that help is not always there. The Internet does not always perform the way it needs to. I think that eventually some of those things will change and we will be able to rely on it more, but today my opinion is that it is not there.

Richard J. Rovinelli, Ph.D. (American Board of Family Practice): I am consulting with one of the divisions at Oracle Software. They are delivering short certification tests to their own employees right now via the Worldwide

Web.They have solved certain security issues for their purposes. People take short tests in short time lines and have to pass a large number of them, so the security problem of someone sitting there with a book in their lap does not particularly bother them. They find the Internet very satisfactory to deliver their tests. The issue, I think, with all of the technology and with all of the methodologies and all of the possibilities is to keep in mind they are tools in a toolbox. You use the tools that help you build what you are trying to build. For the Oracle Software group, delivering their in-house test on the Worldwide Web works fine.

M. Paul Capp, M.D. (American Board of Radiology): We heard from the keynote speaker and other presenters about the potential advantages of the computer. But their comments relate particularly to the current written examinations. In this room, I suspect that of the twenty-four ABMS Member Boards, fifteen still give the oral examination. It would be helpful to give us some input as to the potential substitution of the "computerized examination" for the current oral examination. Most of us (i.e., the fifteen boards that give the oral exam) think that we test something differently by using an oral examination.

Dr. Rovinelli: The project at the American Board of Family Practice initially discussed what kind of additional information can be added to the process of assessing physicians. We were concerned about gaining more information for the recertification process to assess physicians who have been in practice for seven years. We do not know as much about them as we know about physicians who finish residency training immediately before the initial certification. We know how many procedures they have completed and what patients they have seen. We conceptualized the computer project, interestingly enough, as a form of oral examination. It was conceived as a relatively open process in which the physician could ask a series of questions, but eventually the computer could even address issues associated with querying physicians about data. For example, the computer could query on the issue, "Why did you choose that particular differential, can you associate that differential with a particular laboratory finding?" With the advent of expert systems and the tremendous amount of work that continues in expert systems, that indeed will be the future. I agree that oral examinations add something to the process. A number of years ago I had an opportunity to look at the American Board of Radiology's oral examination and I was very impressed. I am also extremely impressed with what the American Board of Psychiatry and Neurology does in their oral examination. But I would be very reluctant to advocate those examinations until we had an adequate mechanism for addressing the kinds of information obtained in those programs. I do think that there is a tremendous possibility for computer-based testing to do just that. Notice that the oral examination does not deal with issues such as procedural or interpersonal skills, factors probably not easily addressed in the computer-based examination.

James M. Woolfenden, M.D. (American Board of Nuclear Medicine): As we look at the possibility of developing a computer-based examination, the prospect is not very appealing having to acquire hardware that would be used once or twice a year for a relatively small number of candidates. Our preference would be to devote the resources to software in the examination itself. Is there some listing, preferably an annotated listing, of resources, sites or centers for computer-based testing? I know that one or two of the exhibitors at the conference provide this service, but is there a more complete listing that might be available?

Dr. Rosen: I am not aware of such a listing. The list of computerized testing vendors today is reasonably short; you could probably collect it from several people here in the room. You need to compare the kinds of networks and the kinds of hardware that are available to you in those systems. I suspect the list is perhaps three or four vendors in all.

Dr. Rovinelli: I'd like to make a comment. Here is an opportunity for specialty boards to look very carefully at cooperation as has been discussed a number of times. Very low volume and very high technical requirements pose problems for commercial vendors. It seems to me that 10 or 15 sites around the country, with each specialty board sponsoring a site, would give an opportunity to put the testing sites in place realistically without the economic impact of each board building their own; or, having to face some of the issues faced by commercial vendors for high quality examinations and low volume of examinees. It is an issue that has to be addressed, clearly, but I think there are solutions and one of them is cooperation.

Stewart B. Dunsker, M.D. (American Board of Neurological Surgery): I enjoyed your presentation and volume certainly is a problem, as just alluded to. At what point would you have reached a number of examinees that would not have been economically feasible for a computer-based examination, and you would have to use paper-and-pencil tests? How do you determine those numbers?

Dr. Rovinelli: That is a question that each board has to ask themselves, in terms of what they want to do with the examination program. If you have reached a point where paper-and-pencil examinations are not producing what you want in terms of assessment of physicians' skills, then it is time to look into using computers. At that point in time, you must address budget issues. Dr. William Hartmann, for example, would be an excellent person to talk to about that specific question. The American Board of Pathology has made a tremendous commitment as an organization to computer-based testing. They probably have volumes of candidates similar to your board. In their particular case they made a decision that it is very important to use computer-based tests, we will do it now, and we will absorb the costs associated with it. Again, I think specialty boards need to be looking seriously and talking with each other in terms of how to share these resources, and how to help in moving toward computer-based testing. I do believe that computer-based assessment is the future. There are forces outside of medicine and psychometrics, for example the use of certification by health maintenance organizations (HMOs), that are pushing specialty boards to look seriously at the viability of continuous daily testing, rather than the traditional format of once a year.

PSYCHOMETRIC ASPECTS OF COMPUTER-BASED TESTING

PART 3

Psychometric Issues in Computer-Based Testing

Alternatives to Current Methods: Decision-Theoretic Approaches

Discussion

Psychometric Issues in Computer-Based Testing

John J. Norcini, Ph.D.
American Board of Internal Medicine

The past twenty years have seen a dramatic increase in the power and use of the computer. Not surprisingly, these developments are beginning to effect the way in which physicians are tested. This paper focuses on three general measurement issues that are essential for making judgments about the quality of a test: reproducibility, equivalence, and validity. For each, the concept will be described in nontechnical terms, its importance will be outlined, and some of the factors influencing it will be presented. Notably absent from this list are scoring and standard-setting. These are important and raise a number of unresolved problems, but they should not be the basis for a decision about whether to proceed.

The remainder of the chapter will focus on four types of computer-based examinations: linear, simulation, adaptive, and continuous practice assessment. Each type will be briefly described, its general advantages and disadvantages will be outlined, with particular attention paid to the reproducibility, equivalence, and validity of the method.

Reproducibility

An important scientific attribute of a laboratory test is its consistency in yielding the same result if the same measurement process is repeated with the same method. This common sense notion applies to educational measures as well. It is important to know that if we gave the same candidates the same test two weeks apart, and they learned nothing in the meantime, they would get the same scores; their results should be reproducible.[1]

53

There are a variety of ways to assess reproducibility and the details are of limited interest for this presentation.[2] However, the concept is crucial in making decisions because it directly influences the number of false positives, i.e., candidates whose true ability is not sufficient for certification, but who pass anyway because of errors of measurement. In fact, the certification process actually maximizes the number of false positives because unqualified candidates have the opportunity to take the test several times and maximize their chances of passing based on measurement errors. If the reproducibility of a test is poor enough, virtually all candidates will pass it after a few tries.

There are a number of factors that influence the reproducibility of scores, ranging from the definition of the domain to be tested through the mechanics of developing the answer key. All are relevant for computer-based testing but four deserve particular attention: *test length, complexity, controversy*, and *redundancy*.

It is widely agreed that physician performance is case specific; performance on one question or case does not predict performance on other cases.[3] Therefore, a test must contain a large number of questions to ensure a stable estimate of ability. All other things being equal, the longer the test, the more reproducible the scores will be.

The second factor influencing reproducibility is *complexity*. Not surprisingly, assessments of complex skills are usually more time consuming than assessment of simple skills. For example, on average it takes longer to establish whether a physician can manage a single patient correctly than whether he or she can read a single ECG correctly. Therefore, tests of simple skills will usually yield more reproducible scores in a fixed amount of testing time than tests of complex skills.[4]

The third factor that influences reproducibility is *controversy*. Variability among experts in defining acceptable performance on the same case adversely affects reproducibility. This variability or controversy is often a product of legitimate differences between experts. Regardless of the source, controversy leads to variability in identification of the correct responses to cases, difficulty in generating the answer key, and therefore, lower reproducibility.[5]

The final factor that influences reproducibility is *redundancy*. Clinical situations often contain a number of redundant cues, some of which are interdependent and most of which point to the same conclusion. Uncontrolled, this inadvertently produces higher scores for examinees whose style of response is to select a number of options or take many actions and this artificially inflates estimates of reproducibility.[4]

Equivalence

Virtually all licensing and certifying bodies administer their tests over time. For many reasons, including security, they need to create different versions or forms of the same test by including some number of new items. If the pass-fail decisions on these tests are not equivalent, it is unfair to candidates who might have been successful had they taken a different version of the test. It is also unacceptable for the public, since it requires them to know when someone was certified or licensed as well as whether they were certified or licensed. In essence, failure to ensure the equivalence of pass-fail decisions undermines the meaning of the certificate and creates *vintages* of certified or licensed specialists.

There are three major factors which influence the equivalence of pass-fail decisions. First, and most important, is *test content*. Different forms of an examination need to test the same medical content in the same proportions. Second, the tests need to perform equally well from a psychometric perspective; they should be of *comparable difficulty and discrimination*. Finally, most licensing and certifying boards use some type of statistical procedure to remove differences in the difficulty of different forms or versions of the test. This is called *equating*; there are many statistical techniques available for this purpose.[6] The only constraint is that the methods used must fit the test data and work well with it.

Validity

The last and probably the most important of the measurement issues described here is validity. As the word implies, validity refers to whether the inferences we draw based on test scores are correct and meaningful.[7] For the ABMS Member Boards, the inference is that candidates have enough knowledge and skill to be able to provide competent care in the specialty. Validation of this inference is an ongoing process and it should include any relevant information or research. Obviously, anything that adversely affects the validity of a test renders the certificate less meaningful.

Numerous factors influence validity, and it is well beyond the scope of this chapter to identify all of them. Instead, I will focus on three issues that have particular relevance to computer-based testing. First, for certification and licensure examinations, *test content* is the most important factor in establishing that the inferences made regarding the scores are correct.[8] Specifically, the content must reflect the practice of the profession. As an aside, the content of training is only tangentially relevant to certification and then it is relevant only to the extent that it reflects practice.

Second in importance is *test security* since prior knowledge of the questions and correct responses would make scores completely meaningless. This threat to validity is of increasing concern as certification becomes more widely used by managed care concerns (or establishments) as a device to reduce the surplus of physicians, especially specialists.

Third is *fidelity*, or the degree to which the test looks and feels real. This is mostly an issue of perception rather than substance, since there is little data supporting the common sense notion that high fidelity tests have better relationships with other markers of competence than low fidelity tests of the same content.[9] However, a high fidelity test is clearly easier to defend than a low fidelity test.

Types of Computer-Based Examinations

For purposes of this chapter, computer-based examinations have been divided into four types: linear examinations, simulations or adapting item content, adapting administration, and continuous practice assessment. This classification scheme is loosely based on work published in the general measurement literature. It has been applied to medicine to provide a convenient way to frame the issues.[10,11] Each of these types of computer-based tests is described and the advantages and disadvantages will be outlined briefly with particular attention to the three measurement issues just presented. A fuller treatment can be found elsewhere.[11]

Linear Computer-Based Examinations

In a linear computer-based examination, the computer administers a test that could otherwise be delivered in a more traditional way. For example, the multiple-choice questions that form the certifying examination of the American Board of Internal Medicine could be put on a computer. Each item would be presented on the screen, candidates would respond by simply pressing a key or pointing and clicking, and all candidates assigned the same form of the test would see the same questions.

There are at least three features of this method of administration that are noteworthy when compared to paper-and-pencil versions of the same test. First, immediate feedback (e.g., scores) can be given to examinees at the end of the test. Second, this type of testing provides access to the computer's capacity for sophisticated display of test materials such as graphics or motion. Third, by eliminating the opportunity to look ahead, computer presentation does away with the effects of cueing and sequencing for item formats where this has been a problem.

In terms of psychometrics, there is clearly not much difference between administration of a linear computer-based examination and a paper-and-pencil version of the same test. The questions are the same and the test forms are the same. Consequently, only minor differences would be expected in reproducibility, equivalence, and most evidence related to validity. However, compared to large group administration with printed material, computer delivery raises an interesting set of security issues.

One of the major security concerns with any test is that candidates will memorize the questions and share them. In many situations, computer-based testing makes this problem worse. There are two general approaches to minimizing it. One approach is to administer the test to everyone at the same time using a large number of computers. The other approach is to administer tests over time with a smaller infrastructure, but drawing on a very large item pool. Either way, it is unlikely to make linear computer-based testing preferable to a written exam. It is not a better measuring device and expensive steps are needed to administer simultaneously or write large numbers of questions.

On the other hand, a strength of computer-based testing, if done properly, is that it helps assure secure delivery of test material to the examining site. Consequently, it may be the best form of testing if there are uncontrollable problems in printing and shipping test books.

Simulations

In simulations, the computer is used to imitate the patient portion of the clinical encounter. The physician manages a computer-based patient as he or she would in real life and the patient responds as a result of the disease process and/or the physician's actions. Unlike linear computer-based testing, the power of the computer is really used. For example, in the National Board of Medical Examiner's clinical case simulations (CBX), the candidate can ask questions, perform a physical examination, obtain laboratory results, prescribe therapies, and the like. After each question, the computer responds as the patient or the laboratory would have. This questioning continues until the candidate reaches a conclusion or the patient status changes. In other simulations, hardware and software are added to the computer to assess procedural skills like endoscopy, physical examination skills and cognitive skills using models like HARVEY, or a cardiac simulation using a manikin.

This methodology has some of the same advantages as linear computerized testing: the possibilities of immediate feedback and sophisticated display. On the other hand, it is time consuming and expensive to develop test materials and scoring algorithms. A large number of interrelated actions need to be specified as part of case writing and weighted as part of scoring. The development of sophisticated case authoring and debugging tools are an important aspect of any practical plan to use simulations.

All other things being equal, simulations yield less reproducible scores per unit of testing time than a multiple-choice question-based examination (MCQ).[4] Each case takes more time to complete than a single MCQ, so candidates get through a smaller number of simulations in the same amount of time. Moreover, because simulations faithfully reproduce the clinical situation, much of what the examinee does is routine or redundant, so getting to the testing point takes considerable time. Finally, simulations capture all of the complexities and controversies in patient care that lead to difficulties in identifying optimal performance.

The issue of limited sampling of cases also makes it more difficult to establish equivalence both in terms of content and performance. After all, if a test consists of 10 or 20 simulations and the domain is relatively broad, like internal medicine, it will be difficult to assure comparable content and difficulty. In addition, the statistical methods used to establish equivalence are less well developed in testing situations where the number of cases is small. There are, however, some promising developments along these lines that require further study.[12]

The limited number of cases in simulations also affects validity because it reduces content coverage. On the other hand, security is enhanced because case disguise should be relatively easy and no single candidate will experience all the pathways through a simulation. Likewise, the test is of higher fidelity and should be more easily defended on grounds of relevance.

Adaptive Tests

Adapting administration or item presentation is similar to simulation in that it uses the computer's intelligence to adapt to an examinee's response. However, the adaptation is psychometrically-based rather than medically-based. The computer software is programmed to estimate the ability of the examinee after each question and then select test items that are targeted to the candidate's ability. This iterative process continues until there is confidence the examinee's level of ability has been determined and a pass/fail decision can be made.[13]

Just as with the other types of computer-based testing, adapting administration has the advantages of immediate feedback and enhanced display of graphic material. Furthermore, each examinee is challenged only by those questions near his or her ability level. Consequently, adaptive tests can yield a 30 percent to 50 percent reduction in testing time over a paper-and-pencil test.

All other things being equal, an adaptive test yields more reproducible scores per unit of testing time than a linear examination. In the latter, the vast majority of the questions a candidate answers are either too easy or too hard. Although they provide some measurement information, they do not make the best use of the testing time available. Consequently, an adaptive test yields a more reproducible pass/fail decision if it is the same length as a linear exam, and equivalent pass/fail decisions with a shorter test.

One of the more challenging aspects of an adaptive test is the fact that virtually all of the candidates are taking different forms of the test. Clearly, equivalence is a major issue. To make adaptive testing work, the items need to meet the strict assumptions of a psychometric model and questions must be available for many different content areas and levels of ability.[13] Not all content domains and items are able to meet these stringent criteria, so adaptive testing is limited somewhat in its scope. On the other hand, when psychometric and model data fit is good and proper content balancing is built into the process, equivalence of pass/fail decisions can be maintained.

Finally, adaptive testing software will, without modification, select items on a psychometric basis without regard to content. To ensure no loss in validity, most test developers have constrained the software to choose from particular content areas so as not to adversely affect validity. This results in a small loss in efficiency, but it ensures that adaptive tests are as appropriate from a content perspective as their linear counterparts. On the other hand, adaptive testing does provide some advantage in terms of security. Candidates take a subset of items and the software can be used to control the amount of item exposure; adaptive tests are thus less vulnerable than linear tests.

Continuous Practice Assessment

Unlike traditional formal testing, continuous practice assessment relies on patients or items that are part of the daily activities of physicians.[14] Evaluation of the outcomes of these patients or the process of care constitutes the method of assessment. For instance, the medical records of a single physician could be abstracted for information about the process of care and how well his or her patients were doing, or such information could be derived from the large databases being constructed now by many managed care organizations. The computer is a key piece of this method because the amount of information needed is too great to process otherwise.

This method provides an assessment of actual performance rather than of the potential to perform, and it is tailored to the activities of the test taker. In addition, it is generally unobtrusive and provides the groundwork for constant, helpful feedback that could have a positive impact on patient care. However, the vast majority of the research has been done in hospital settings where patients are acutely ill and surgical procedures are involved. This is in contrast to the ambulatory setting where problems are chronic, good outcomes are difficult to define, and significant follow-up is required to document an effect. Moreover, most of the research in this area has been done with a limited number of conditions using large groups of physicians. Considerable work on the psychometric characteristics of this method still remains before it will be useful in the evaluation of the individual practitioner.

In most content areas, assessments of the outcomes of a large number of patients are required to obtain a reproducible estimate of physician performance. For example, data developed by the American Board of Internal Medicine suggest that 30-50 patients are needed for a stable assessment of patient satisfaction.[15] These results suggest that it is feasible to assess the outcomes of care only for common problems, since these will be the only areas where reasonable estimates of individual performance can be obtained.

Equivalence is one of the biggest problems with continuous assessment. Case mix and severity of illness clearly vary by physician. Moreover, an individual physician is not the sole cause of any particular outcome. The patient's willingness and ability to comply with the doctor's orders, the resources available, the performances of other members of the health care team, and a host of other factors also contribute. Initial work in controlling for some of these factors is underway, but the methods have not yet reached the level of precision necessary for certification.[16]

In terms of validity, assessment of patient outcomes is clearly superior to other methods in that it is an actual assessment of performance. It has no issues of security and the only limitation relates to the privacy of patient information and the fact that it is unlikely to provide a good assessment of infrequent but important problems.

Summary

To summarize, there are three important measurement issues that influence the decisions to pursue computer-based testing: reproducibility—will candidates get the same score if given the same examination again; equivalence—will candidates get the same score if given a different form of the examination; and validity—are we making appropriate inferences based on the scores.

Four types of computer-based examinations are compared along the three measurement issues. Linear computer-based tests are basically the same as traditional written examinations in terms of reproducibility, equivalence, and validity; security may be a concern depending on the circumstances. Simulations have some problems with reproducibility and equivalence but have advantages in terms of security and fidelity. The strengths of adaptive test administration include reproducibility and security. However, use of this technology requires a strong psychometric model that is not equally applicable to all medical content. Finally, continuous practice assessment currently has serious limitations in terms of reproducibility and equivalence but the validity of the assessments made with this form of evaluation is outstanding.

This is an exciting time to be involved in evaluation. It is my belief that the computer will be the dominant tool in the assessment of physicians within the next decade.

References

1. Brennan RL. *Elements of generalizability theory.* ACT Publications: Iowa City, Iowa, 1983.

2. Crocker L, Algina J. *Introduction of classical and modern test theory.* Holt, Rinehart, Winston: New York, 1986.

3. Elstein AS, Shulman LS, Sprafka SA. *An analysis of clinical reasoning.* Cambridge, Mass.: Harvard Press, 1978.

4. Norcini JJ, Swanson DB. Factors influencing testing time requirements for written simulations. *Int J Teach Learn Med* 1989; 1:985-91.

5. Norcini JJ. The answer key as a source of error in examinations for professionals. *J Educ Meas* 1987; 24:321-331.

6. Shea JA, Norcini JJ. Equating. In Impara, JC (Ed.), *Licensure testing: Purposes, procedures, and practices.* Lincoln, Nebraska: Buros Institute of Mental Measurement, 1995.

7. Wainer H, Braun HI. *Test validity.* Lawrence Erlbaum: Hillsdale, New Jersey: 1988.

8. Kane MT. The validity of licensure examinations. *Amer Psychologist* 1982; 37:911-918.

9. Swanson DB, Norcini JJ, Grosso LJ. Assessment of clinical competence: Written and computer-based simulations. *Assess Eval Higher Educ* 1987; 12:220-246.

10. Bunderson CV, Inouye DK, Olsen JB. The four generations of computerized educational measurement. In Linn, R.L. (Ed.) *Educational Meas.* New York: Macmillan, 1989.

11. Norcini JJ. Computers in physician licensure and certification: New methods of assessment. *J Educ Computing* 1994; 10:161-171.

12. Norcini JJ. Equivalent pass/fail decisions. *J Educ Meas* 1990; 27:59-66.

13. Wainer H. *Computerized adaptive testing: A primer.* Hillsdale, New Jersey: Lawrence Erlbaum, 1990.

14. Kremer BK. Physician recertification and outcomes assessment. *Eval Hlth Prof* 1991; 14:187-200.

15. Swanson DB, Webster GD, Norcini JJ. Precision of patient ratings of residents' humanistic qualities: How many items and patients are enough? In W Bender, CM Metz, HJ Van Rossum (Eds.) *Proceedings of the third international conference on teaching and assessing clinical competence,* 1989.

16. Iezzoni L. Measuring the severity of illness and case mix. In N Goldfield and DB Nash (Eds.) *Providing quality care: The challenge to clinicians.* Philadelphia, Pennsylvania: American College of Physicians, 1989.

Alternatives to Current Methods: Decision-Theoretic Approaches

Charles P. Friedman, Ph.D.
and
Stephen M. Downs, M.D.
University of North Carolina

To make an explicit segue between Dr. John Norcini's paper and this one, we refer to the several "promising developments" he mentioned that require further study. We will introduce a decision-theoretic scoring model for clinical simulations as one of the potentially promising developments and one that requires further study.

Our point of departure is the general problem of scoring clinical simulations. This problem has been around for a long time.[1] One of the challenges is obtaining useful scoring information from a simulated case that goes meaningfully beyond a binary, one or zero score, for each case. After the examinee has spent perhaps half an hour on a simulated case, how can we say more than he or she was right or wrong? If such binary information is the maximum that can be derived from one case, a whole case becomes analogous to one item on a multiple-choice test. A test with a given number of simulations will have a reproducibility comparable to that of a multiple-choice test with a like number of items, and clearly that is a very inefficient way to assess clinical competence. Our goal, therefore, is to obtain more useful scoring information than a binary one or zero score from an exercise which occupies a great amount of examinee time and should, to justify its use in testing, produce additional useful information.

This work is supported by Grant R01-LM-04843 from the National Library of Medicine

Three main points will be addressed. We will:

1. Describe how decision-theoretic techniques can be used for scoring simulations.
2. Discuss possible advantages and disadvantages of this method.
3. Describe a research project under way to investigate decision-theoretic scoring.

The latest information technology, as Dr. Michael Ackerman made very clear in his presentation (see Part 1), will enable us to create and deliver very high fidelity clinical simulations. This is challenging and tantalizing to all of us. The technology is available to process natural language information requests, to allow cases to evolve realistically over time, and to present clinical findings using multimedia. This is not vaporware; the technology to do these things exists today. Furthermore, the problem that has puzzled many people for years—how to avoid the labor intensive and very expensive process of hand authoring the clinical script for each simulated case—may be addressed by techniques whereby cases are generated automatically out of a knowledge base. But, even within the framework of these new developments and the promise of automated case generation, it is still not clear how these cases can be scored. Do the scores one might generate out of a record of how students progress through a case, over fifteen or twenty or thirty minutes of work, tell us anything more about competence than can be obtained from existing methods of testing and scoring? We do not yet know.

Our decision-theoretic approach is based on a rigorous probabilistic model of a clinical problem using a technique known as influence diagrams.[2] For this purpose, we define a problem as a presenting syndrome which could have a wide range of causes. Although most of our work has been in the domain of infectious diseases, the method applies across the spectrum of disease presentations and etiologies. Examples of problems in the domain we have studied include cellulitis, urethritis and pneumonia.

A probabilistic model expresses, among other things, the probability of the presence of specific findings for each of a set of diseases that may be causing the problem, the probability that the patient has one of those specific diseases, and, very important, the utility or value of diagnosing each possible disease conditioned on which disease the patient actually has. As much as possible, although it is not possible to do this entirely, the quantitative relationships that are captured in the model are based on verified medical knowledge. This is, in effect, an "evidence based" approach to the problem of scoring simulations.

Figure 1 shows a piece of a probabilistic model for cellulitis.

Figure 1

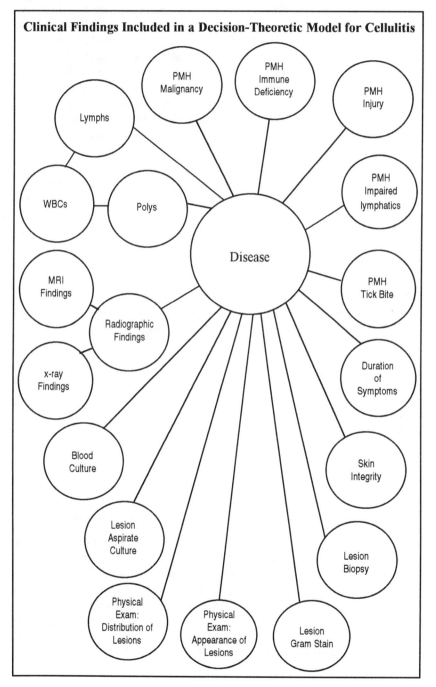

Clinical Findings Included in a Decision-Theoretic Model for Cellulitis

There are about 20 findings associated with the set of possible diseases that could cause cellulitis, as shown in the figure. Our model for cellulitis also includes 14 possible causes (diseases) ranging from common cellulitis to lyme disease and erythema nodosum. Another part of the model not shown in Figure 1, the utility matrix, assigns a value to *concluding* that the patient has one of these 14 diseases, given that the patient *actually* has a particular disease. To cover all possible combinations, the utility matrix for the cellulitis model is 14-by-14. In Table 1 we illustrate a smaller utility matrix for the clinical problem of a skin lesion modeled as having three possible causes. The utility matrix can take into account, for example, that all incorrect diagnoses are not equally incorrect. An incorrect diagnosis resulting in a treatment that would also treat the actual disease would not be nearly as severe a mistake as an incorrect diagnosis which would result in further progression of the patient's disease. Also notice that the utility assigned to correct a diagnosis of malignancy is lower than the utility assigned to correct a diagnosis of pyoderma or tularemia. This builds into the model a representation of the intrinsic severity of the disease or the prognosis attached to actually having that disease. This feature of the model has important implications for scoring simulations that will be addressed later.

Table 1

Example Utility Matrix for a Skin Lesion

		Dz		
		Pyoderma	Malignancy	Tularemia
	Pyoderma	1	0	0.8
Dx	Malignancy	0.95	0.65	0.75
	Tularemia	0.98	0	.9

Dx = Diagnosis made by examinee
Dz = Disease the simulated patient actually has

To see how the scoring mechanism actually works, we will begin with a diagram of a basic clinical simulation (Figure 2). In a simulation the examinee is given very basic and usually minimal information about a presenting problem. The examinee then engages a cycle which consists of requests for clinical findings and obtaining results, cycling through this process as many times either as allowed or as the examinee chooses. Upon emerging from the cycle, the examinee enters a diagnosis which may be correct or incorrect. Real simulations are more complicated,[3] but these basic elements are shared by virtually all simulations.

Figure 2

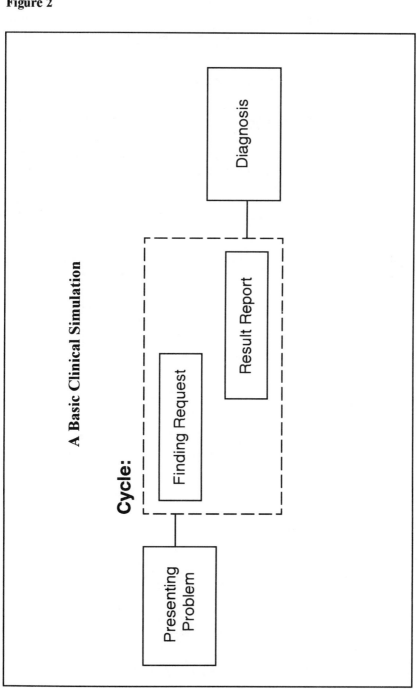

A Basic Clinical Simulation

To attach a scoring model, we feed information about the examinee's progress through the simulation to a decision-theoretic model, as shown in Figure 3. The model is represented as an influence diagram for the clinical problem that is the subject of the simulation. Recall that this clinical problem can be caused by any number of a set of possible diseases, one of which is the correct diagnosis for the particular simulated case the examinee is working. Also as shown in Figure 3 the decision model includes:

1. The utility of making any one of the diagnoses in the set given that the patient has a specific disease $[U(D_x|D_z)]$.

2. The probability of each set of clinical findings being present given that the patient actually has a specific disease $[p(F|D_z)]$.

3. The initial probability $[p(D_z)]$ of each disease for the presenting problem.

More complex influence diagrams may contain more information; but these three sets of quantities are the minimum. It should be emphasized that the decision-theoretic model is a representation of a clinical problem. The model covers many possible clinical presentations of many possible diseases, and is unrelated to any examinees' actual performance on simulated cases.

Figure 3

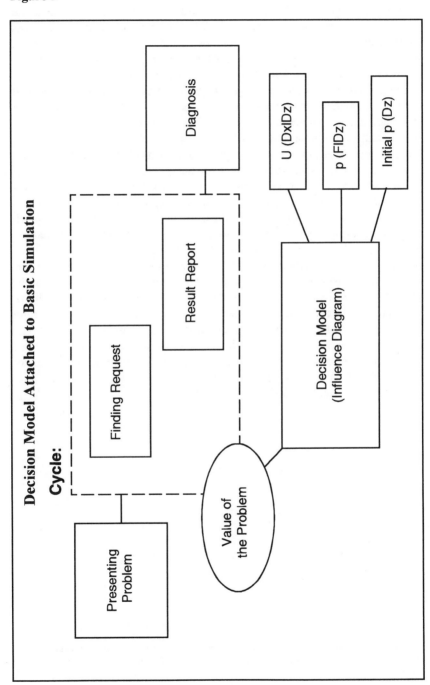

Decision Model Attached to Basic Simulation

Cycle:

Using the information in the model and coupling it to the examinee's trajectory through the problem, the influence diagram can be solved to generate the "expected utility" for each of the possible diagnoses. The optimal diagnosis based on the decision model, at any point in the simulation, is the diagnosis with maximum expected utility. The "value of the problem" as a whole is the expected utility of the optimal diagnosis. It is possible, based on the clinical findings the examinee actually has obtained at any point in the simulation, for the optimal decision not to be the correct diagnosis. This occurs when the particular clinical information the examinee has requested is information that suggests, according to the model, a different diagnosis than the one which is correct. Under some circumstances, an examinee who has partial information about a simulated case *should* be considering diagnoses which are not correct.

So how is scoring information obtained from the model, given an examinee's progression through a simulated case?* One method is to compute the expected value, based on the decision model, of each item of clinical information (each finding) the examinee requests as he or she progresses through the simulation. To do this, we first use the decision model to compute the "value of the problem" before a given information request. After the examinee requests a particular finding, the decision model once again is invoked and computes the value of the problem after the request is made. The difference between these values, as shown in Figure 4, is the expected value of one item of requested information. To obtain an overall index of performance on the entire simulated case, we could compute the average expected value of all clinical findings obtained by the examinee during the progress through a case. Hypothetically, the examinee's selection of findings which have greater expected values should be indicative of higher level performance on the simulation.

---

*Indices similar to these, but computed somewhat differently, as used in the scoring of simulations generated by the ILIAD™ system, a product of Applied Medical Informatics, Inc. of Salt Lake City, Utah.

Figure 4

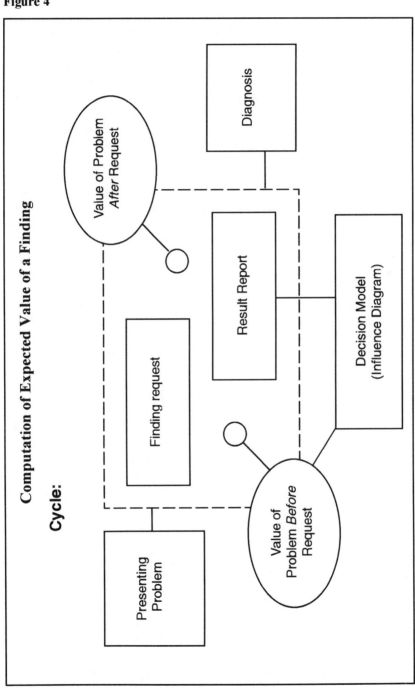

Computation of Expected Value of a Finding

Cycle:

Another element of potentially useful scoring information that can be obtained using the decision-theoretic model relates to the examinee's final diagnosis: the diagnosis he or she makes at the conclusion of working on the simulated case. For example, the model allows us to compute the ratio of the expected utility of the examinee's final diagnosis to the value of the problem (the expected utility of the best diagnosis) at whatever point the final diagnosis is made. If the examinee's final diagnosis is the best diagnosis based on the clinical findings he or she has obtained, this ratio will be 1. If the examinee's diagnosis is sub-optimal, the value of this ratio will be a number greater than zero and less than 1. This number can be used as a scoring index, giving the examinee partial credit for a partially correct diagnosis.

These two scoring indices—(1) average expected value of clinical findings and (2) proportional expected utility of the final diagnosis—have some appealing features. The first index potentially rewards efficiency of information gathering in a simulation. Earlier research on simulations showed that methods which assigned a fixed score to each finding selected by an examinee, independent of the other findings the examinee had already selected, failed to reward the efficiency of experts who were able to come to accurate diagnoses based on much less information than novices required.[4] Such scoring schemes rewarded those who were methodical, and possibly even redundant, in their information gathering as opposed to those who were focused and parsimonious. The second index potentially addresses the equally perplexing problem of how to give an appropriate level of partial credit for incorrect diagnoses. Intuitively, all wrong answers are not equally wrong. Crediting examinees with the expected utility of their final diagnosis, as a fraction of the expected utility of the best diagnosis, may be a useful way to address this problem.

However appealing they may be at an intuitive level, the empirical question that remains before us is whether these decision-theoretic metrics are incrementally valid: whether they add any information beyond what we can get from traditional scoring procedures for simulation. If they do—and this must be studied—consider what might be some of the possible advantages. First, with decision-theoretic methods, scoring can be completely automated. An automated scoring process would not require a human observer or judge to directly evaluate each examinee's pathway through the simulation. Second, once a decision model is developed for a general clinical problem which has many possible causes, all simulations of that problem can be scored using the same decision model. A very large number of cases can be scored using one model.

For example, if a given clinical problem has fifteen plausible items in the differential diagnosis, any clinical case in that problem area, with the true diagnosis being any of the 15 items in the differential, can be scored with the same model. Some problem areas may require more sophisticated models than those we have shown. Interdependencies of tests and costs of obtaining clinical data can be factored into the scoring model.

Third, the entire scoring model is externalized from the specifics of any particular simulated case, and can be applied consistently across these cases. The model takes into account and compensates for the fact that some cases in the problem area may be more difficult than others. An examinee's score is based on how that examinee performed relative to what is optimal for that case. Fourth, objective medical data pertinent to the problem area are the bases for deciding what is optimal. Disease prevalence statistics and probabilities of positive findings in each disease can be culled from the biomedical literature. Although utilities are more intrinsically subjective, the decision-theoretic literature reports several standard methods for obtaining utility estimates. These methods provide confidence that a useful scoring system based, in part, on utilities can be developed.

Fifth and last, decision-theoretic scoring is harmonious with the efforts of several testing agencies to generate simulated cases out of a knowledge base that is already in a decision-theoretic format. In such instances, the decision-theoretic scoring system becomes a direct by-product of the same methodology that is used to create the simulations themselves. The scoring methodology is obtained for free, or nearly free.

Those are some of the potential advantages. What are the potential questions and concerns? As mentioned earlier, utilities are subjective. The 3-by-3 matrix of utilities shown in Table 1 gives a sense of the potential for experts to disagree about the expected utility of each outcome represented as the utility of diagnosing Disease X when the patient actually has Disease Y. It may be that this scoring method will not be generalizable beyond the particular group who quantifies these utilities. A second concern is that efficiency will motivate those creating the scoring models to minimize the number of diagnoses and findings they include. There is countervailing pressure to make the clinical simulations themselves more realistic by maximizing the number of possible diagnoses and clinical findings examinees may consider. We do not yet know if there is a middle ground wherein the problems are simple enough to be modelled but yet complex enough that they can be made into simulations that examinees will find realistic. Third, disease prevalences and other parameters used in decision models may vary regionally or temporally. It may be that the models used to score simulations will "decay" over time or that models which are validated in New York City are not valid in Seattle or Albuquerque. This is a problem that will have to be explored.

Having listed some possible advantages and shortcomings of decision-theoretic simulation scoring, it is important to reemphasize the key question of incremental validity. All who have ventured into the minefield of simulation scoring must remain mindful that the indices generated by decision-theoretic scoring may not provide meaningful information. They may not tell us anything more than existing scoring methods. Or, they may not tell us anything more than a simple binary 1/0 score obtainable simply by determining whether the examinee made the correct diagnosis.

We are in the process now of developing models and simulations for specific problem areas in the general domain of infectious disease. We have developed simulations and models for scoring them in the areas of cellulitis, meningitis, urethritis, and pneumonia. We plan to study the reproducibility and validity of scores generated using the decision-theoretic methods. Data will be provided by third-year medical students and more experienced physicians who complete sets of simulations in these problem areas.

Another project goal is to explore the effect of providing access to biomedical knowledge as part of the simulation environment. We will consider whether an appropriate way to deliver clinical simulations in the future is one that makes access to knowledge resources a routine part of the testing environment. If examinees have access to knowledge resources, the problems are testing not just what is in the examinee's own head but the extent to which the examinee can augment his/her own knowledge with appropriate access to knowledge resources available in electronic form. We will also explore whether our decision-theoretic models can predict when examinees provided with knowledge resources will choose to access them. When the decision model that is tracking an examinee's progress through a case suggests that the examinee should be confused, does the examinee actually feel confused and seek help from an external source?

To revisit our main points, we have described how it might be possible to use decision-theoretic models to score clinical simulations. We have highlighted some potential advantages and disadvantages of these methods. It appears that the most benefit from decision-theoretic scoring stands to be derived if specialty boards and other testing agencies move toward automated generation of simulated cases, using representations of medical knowledge that already are in decision-theoretic form. Under these circumstances, the scoring system comes at a very low incremental cost. We believe that the biggest potential disadvantage of decision-theoretic scoring is the subjectivity inherent in the utility estimates, but that remains to be seen. We are conducting research to explore the incremental validity of decision-theoretic scoring. Within a year, we expect to be able to report some results and will know more about the usefulness of these new approaches for assessment.

References

1. Swanson DB, Norcini JJ, Grosso LJ. Assessment of clinical competence: written and computer-based simulations. *Assess Eval Higher Educ*, 1987;12:220-246.

2. Shachter RD. Evaluating influence diagrams. *Operations Res*, 1986;34:871-82.

3. Friedman CP. Anatomy of the clinical simulation. *Acad Med*, 1995;70:205-208.

4. Newble DI, Hoare J, Baxter A. Patient management problems: Issues of validity. *Med Educ*, 1982;16:137-42.

Discussion

Gerald P. Whelan, M.D. (American Board of Emergency Medicine): Most of what you presented Dr. Friedman had to do with diagnosis. I have two questions. The first is, can you apply the same kind of theoretical models to therapeutic interventions?

Charles P. Friedman, Ph.D. (University of North Carolina): Yes, absolutely. I presented a very basic model, but you can assign utilities and other decision-theoretic attributes to therapies as well as by fairly direct extensions of the same basic method.

Dr. Whelan: The second question is, have you looked at a theoretical approach to the feedback loop of how interventions alter the scenario? Thus, depending on the intervention, the patient's condition changes, or fails to change?

Dr. Friedman: We have thought about this, but obviously the greater the complexity in the simulation, the more the complexity must adhere to the model used to score the simulation. All of this is theoretically possible, although the combination begins to become daunting as you think about assigning numbers to derive conditional possibilities. It becomes a very challenging task to model all these possibilities, but it is possible. The question really is, what is practical?

John R. Hayes, M.D. (St. Vincent Hospital, Indianapolis): I think it is true that the conceptual problems relative to the last question probably are much less important than the time and money ones. I find that encouraging rather than

75

discouraging, because I think it will simply be a matter of time before those almost infinite combinations can be mapped out and used. But, I wanted to suggest to you that the subjectivity about which you are worried, doesn't seem to me to be the largest of the problems that you listed. One of the historical concerns about an oral examination in which an examiner presents a theoretical case which the candidate then discusses is that there can be grotesque differences in the utilities assigned from examiner to examiner. I am a psychiatrist, and nowhere is it more true than in psychiatry where theoretical underpinnings may influence the examiner. In the simulation model you presented the subjective biases for the derivation of the utilities and the utilities are applied to each candidate in the same way. It would be as if a thousand candidates could be examined by the same oral examiner. If he were an "analyst" instead of a "behaviorist," would he in fact derive the same utilities and apply those same biases in exactly the same subjective ways to even out the biases amongst the candidates? I wonder if you could comment on that?

Dr. Friedman: Well, I am delighted that you are less worried about this than I am. In your conference packet there is an example of an actual problem worked out in detail, the pyoderma tularemia malignancy case. I think if you look at that example, you will see the sensitive issues in scoring. For example, based on its expected value, what is the best hypothesis to consider at a given point in the case relative to the actual values in that utility matrix? When I look at numbers like those in the utility matrix, I get concerned that a little wiggle, a little bit of measurement error in effect, might dramatically affect how someone will perform on the case. I am more sanguine about the ability of expert panels deciding and other methods of using experts, and using standard decision-theoretic techniques for listing utilities to derive numbers that everybody will basically accept. As you point out, once those numbers have been calculated, they will be applied consistently by the scoring algorithm. What concerns me, when I put on my psychometric hat, is the almost non-linearity of the utilities and the sensitivity of results to measurement error.

William H. Hartmann, M.D. (American Board of Pathology): Dr. Norcini, I want to congratulate you on your presentation and the reality that it brought to the session. Do you have any feeling about the relationship between the computer models of the examinations that you described and whether or not those are evolutionary stages in computer testing entirely separated from each other, or related by the circumstance of testing?

John J. Norcini, Ph.D. (American Board of Internal Medicine): I think that all those methods will actually merge at some point down the line. I do not see any reason why there cannot be an adaptive test with simulations. I expect that within five or ten years they will all merge and look like one way of doing testing.

PLANNING SUCCESSFUL CONVERSIONS TO COMPUTER-BASED EXAMINATIONS

PART 4

Overview of a Successful Conversion

Certifying Boards and Computer-Based Examinations

Candidates and Computer-Based Examinations

Discussion

Overview of a Successful Conversion

Anthony R. Zara, Ph.D.
National Council of State Boards of Nursing

The National Council of State Boards of Nursing (National Council) administers the national nurse licensure examinations, NCLEX-RN™ (for registered nurses) and NCLEX-PN™ (for practical nurses), nationally to almost 200,000 candidates annually. In 1987, the National Council of State Boards of Nursing initiated a project to investigate the feasibility of administering the NCLEX using computerized adaptive testing (CAT). As of April 1, 1994, the NCLEX was converted from a standard paper-and-pencil administration format to CAT. This transition was accomplished over approximately seven years and included: a pilot test of the software, a set of operational and psychometric field tests, and an extensive national beta test (with over 9,000 participants). This paper outlines the conditions under which this successful transition occurred and presents the planning process and key issues addressed by the National Council.

Determine the Baseline Environment
Leading to the Computer-Based Exam

In order to plan successfully the transition from an existing paper-and-pencil examination process to a computer-based process, it is important to determine *a priori* the organizational motivations for thinking about this change, who are the players that can affect the process, and what resources can be brought to bear in making it happen. For our project, the National Council reviewed the existing paper-and-pencil process and determined that computerized adaptive testing offered many potential benefits for a national licensure testing program.

From the beginning of the research, important benefits were anticipated for both candidates and boards of nursing. Candidates are able to take the NCLEX in a quiet, private, and self-paced environment. Examinations can be scheduled year-round, enabling them to take the test closer to graduation or the time they wish to begin practice. Results are made available to candidates much sooner than for the paper-and-pencil administration: the normal turnaround time since CAT adoption can be measured in weeks rather than months after test administration.

Boards of nursing have also benefited from using CAT to administer NCLEX. Rather than being responsible for obtaining facilities and proctors for two yearly mass administrations per examination, the NCLEX is administered by a professional testing service. The NCLEX utilizes unique sets of items for each candidate (using CAT), preventing the possibility of a "test form" being compromised since there is no single test form administered at any particular time. Thus, the integrity of the NCLEX is better protected, even though administration is scheduled daily. The CAT examination process has the advantage of better precision of measurement for each individual examinee when making pass/fail decisions, rather than providing a group-based reliability estimate. Enhanced reliability enables boards of nursing to better fulfill their mandate to protect the public health, safety, and welfare by licensing only competent individuals. The immediate scoring has greatly reduced the waiting time from NCLEX administration to receipt of results, and boards of nursing can reduce the amount of time that graduate nurse candidates are able to practice through the use of temporary permits. It also speeds up the identification of individuals not ready to enter practice. Since test booklets are no longer printed, the availability of questions in hard copy form has been drastically reduced. In addition, opportunities for candidates to copy answers from other test takers during the examination have been virtually eliminated.

Plan for Necessary Psychometric Foundations

After the organizational analysis concluded that CAT was the preferred computerized testing modality for the National Council, significant planning was necessary to assure that the required psychometric foundations for CAT were attainable by the NCLEX program, including the properties required by item response theory (IRT, see e.g., Hambleton & Swaminathan).[1] The National Council has a strong organizational mandate to develop high quality licensure examinations and the lure of CAT's benefits could not be allowed to compromise the NCLEX program's psychometric soundness or legal defensibility.

One of the most important considerations in the transition to a CAT examination program is test items and the size of the item pools. Most of the common CAT models require a "large" IRT-calibrated item pool as a prerequisite. Because of the National Council's history of extensive NCLEX development work for the paper-and-pencil version, there were large numbers of

NCLEX items already available and IRT-calibrated (using the Rasch model).[2] The National Council also conducted a study to estimate the number of items needed to support year-round CAT testing. Important variables considered in developing the estimate were: (1) acceptable item exposure rates, (2) acceptable item overlap across candidates, (3) the distribution of candidate competence, and (4) the distribution of item difficulties.

Depending on the computerized testing model under consideration, it may be important to consider the psychometric nature of the construct being measured. Given the strong assumptions of IRT, it was important for National Council to demonstrate that entry-level nursing competence (as measured by the NCLEX) could function as a unidimensional construct. National Council conducted a series of research studies (with CTB/McGraw-Hill) to investigate the dimensionality of the NCLEX. It was determined that NCLEX items functioned sufficiently in a single dimension and met this assumption for IRT use.

Other decisions influenced by psychometric data need to be considered when planning a transition to computerized testing. The specific nature of the examination items can be important for a number of reasons. Given the right conditions, the unique properties of using a computer to administer a test have been shown to be inconsequential in the testing process. Hofer and Green[3] support the equivalence of paper-and-pencil and computer testing modes when using multiple-choice items not dealing with sensitive or personally-threatening issues. Research by Kiely, Zara, and Weiss[4] supports the equivalence of computer and paper-and-pencil administered multiple-choice items which do not contain extremely long text passages. With the IRT-based CAT modality, it was important for the NCLEX items to be locally independent.[1] Based on some earlier research conducted to determine the performance characteristics of cased-based items versus "stand-alone" items in the paper-and-pencil NCLEX, the National Council had begun to develop only "stand-alone" items for several years prior to the transition to CAT. Stand-alone items refer to those examination questions that consist of simply a question stimulus and the response choices. This construction is in contrast to case-based items, which consist of a narrative background of case information, question stimulus, and response choices. Case-based items are usually constructed so that one case narrative is attached to several questions. Research was also conducted to determine whether the splitting of case-based items into stand-alone items would have any adverse effect on the item's measurement properties. The research showed that splitting case-based NCLEX items into stand-alone items did not affect their measurement qualities and that long case-based item sets could be separated and formatted to fit completely onto the computer screen (without the need for scrolling text).

Determine Necessary Decision-Making Processes for the Organization

Many of the issues in preparing to convert to CAT from a traditional paper-and-pencil administered high-stakes licensure examination are technical in nature, and the principal participants are often measurement experts (rather than organizationally-savvy staff). Sometimes it is difficult to focus sufficient organizational attention and resources on the key factors to a successful conversion. For these reasons it is very important to identify the important stakeholders and their decision-making influence on the examination program early in the planning process. Typical stakeholders in licensure are board members, candidates, educators, legislators, the public, staff, committee members. Depending on the organization and the examination program, stakeholder groups will differ in amounts of decision-making power (the capability to hinder or facilitate the process) at various times during the transition.

Once the universe of stakeholders is identified, ensuring decision-maker and other stakeholder buy-in is imperative. Even the most technologically advanced, benefit-rich, and cost-effective program can fail for lack of strong supporters. The National Council was able to develop wide-spread support by first determining the effects of the change to CAT on the various stakeholders, then emphasizing the importance of the beneficial effects, and consistently acknowledging and trying to mitigate the negative effects.

Once benefits of the conversion are acknowledged by stakeholders, there may be pressure to accelerate the project pace, making it difficult to allow sufficient time to complete the necessary preparation and provide the full information necessary for constructive decision making. The National Council avoided this temptation, and was careful to pace the project's deliverables and decision-making so that time was available should any unanticipated problems be uncovered during the research and development activities. Another strategy that worked well to facilitate the decision-making was the National Council's practice of open and early communications about the project to all stakeholders.

Boards of Nursing

The 62 U.S. boards of nursing were targeted as primary stakeholders, since the National Council of State Boards of Nursing is an association of the state boards whose mission is to provide services to the boards, the primary product being the NCLEX. In the National Council's governance structure the Delegate Assembly (made up of two representatives from each board) is the ultimate policy-making body of the organization. Reflecting this decision-making structure, the CAT feasibility research was separated into two phases, an affirmative Delegate Assembly decision being needed to continue into the second phase. The issues important to boards included state law and administrative rule changes needed prior to CAT implementation, costs to boards for administering CAT, candidate costs, staffing patterns, state nursing board computer needs, item pool security, administration site issues, and internal workflow procedures.

Many of the boards' concerns over the change in administration method were alleviated through the bidding process for acquiring a test service. The Delegate Assembly discussed the options and determined that the NCLEX would be administered by a professional test service. The paper-and-pencil NCLEX was administered by the nursing boards. This Delegate Assembly decision effectively ended boards' concerns about administration costs to boards, questions about numbers of computers needed, board security issues, and administration staffing needs. The security plans subsequently developed by the selected vendors, Educational Testing Service (ETS) and Sylvan Learning Systems (Sylvan), in consultation with the National Council, provided reassurance that the item pools and data transfer procedures would be appropriately safeguarded.

Even with their administration concerns addressed, boards of nursing still had to make many changes in order to prepare for the CAT administration of NCLEX. In about half of the states and territories, state laws and/or administrative rules had to be changed to allow for CAT administration of NCLEX. The National Council provided assistance by developing and disseminating suggested wording changes to the previously distributed *Model Nursing Practice Act*[5] and *Model Nursing Administrative Rules.*[6] The National Council also provided on-site assistance to boards needing help in understanding what CAT administration of NCLEX meant with respect to their existing state laws and rules.

The issues of board of nursing workflow were addressed throughout the transition process in a number of ways. First, the National Council made a commitment to supply each board of nursing with its own PC-based computer system to communicate with ETS/Sylvan and the National Council for NCLEX-related issues. Next, ETS developed a software package (Member Board Office System or MBOS) for boards of nursing to communicate candidate eligibility, receive results, and create a state-based candidate database. The NCLEX Beta Test provided the State Boards an opportunity to conduct hands-on practice in using the new data transfer and communications software. The National Council has also supplied a powerful electronic mail system, which enabled each board of nursing to be connected with other boards, the National Council, ETS, and Sylvan.

Candidates and Educators

The group most personally affected by the change in NCLEX administration from paper-and-pencil to CAT are the candidates for nurse licensure who must all take the examination as one requirement. Although candidates and educators have no actual decision-making responsibility with boards of nursing or the

National Council, their understanding and acceptance of CAT was important for developing an overall positive stakeholder attitude about the conversion. Their resistance to the project would have made boards more hesitant in deciding to implement CAT and may have stopped it completely.

Throughout the seven years of the research and conversion, the National Council was sensitive to the effects of the administrative changes and made major efforts to communicate the impact of CAT. Because students are a difficult population to reach directly, the National Council also worked hard to communicate the changes in NCLEX and the benefits to candidates of CAT to educators, employers, and review courses. Brochures, a series of custom videos, speaking opportunities, and many other methods were used to disseminate information. The National Council and ETS/Sylvan worked together to develop a "practice disk" that provides general information about CAT, information about the Sylvan testing centers, and provided example test questions to practice using the two-key NCLEX computer interface. All three groups made a commitment to provide this diskette as widely as possible at no cost to the user.

Critical Issues in Decision-Making

As the National Council progressed through the CAT Feasibility Study (Phase I and Phase II research) and through the full-scale transition to CAT, there were several critical time periods when the organizational decision makers needed to determine the direction of the project. At these junctures it was very important for staff and the involved committees to provide the Board of Directors and Delegate Assembly with the information necessary to make these key decisions. Where the "continue vs. kill the project" decisions were made and when service expectations were developed, were instrumental in shaping the final program.

Information on psychometric, legal, and operational decisions. During the Feasibility Study, it was necessary to develop detailed information about the effects of CAT on the NCLEX. Phase I activities mainly consisted of developing and pilot testing CAT software on nurses and determining whether they could use the computer to take an examination. Phase I outcomes showed that nurses could use the computer and that previous computer experience did not affect their results. After evaluating the results of Phase I, the Delegate Assembly voted to continue the project into Phase II.

The goals of Phase II were to obtain detailed information on the feasibility of using CAT by investigating operational issues, test security, legal issues, and the psychometric equivalence of CAT-administered and the paper-and-pencil administered NCLEX. The National Council's decision to implement CAT was based largely on the psychometric, operational, and security results from two national, large-scale field tests with registered nurses conducted during July, 1990 and February, 1991. The CAT field testing was conducted in conjunction with the standard NCLEX-RN in four states during each administration using a pre- and post-test counterbalanced design. The CAT examinations were scheduled within a two-week period either before or after the normal NCLEX-RN examination to assure that the candidate preparation levels were roughly the same for NCLEX and CAT. Field testing for the NCLEX-PN was conducted in October 1992.

The CAT field test examinations were composed of test items drawn from a sample of approximately 3,000 items in the NCLEX-RN item pool. Each candidate's CAT items were selected to conform to the *NCLEX-RN Test Plan* (see e.g., Kingsbury & Zara[7] for an explanation of constrained CAT item selection). The CAT exams administered a maximum of 300 and minimum of 60 items, with the exact number dependent on the candidate's test performance. Candidates with scores close to the pass/fail cut score were administered more items; those far from the cut score (either above or below) took fewer items before the CAT software was able to make an accurate pass/fail decision. The paper-and-pencil examinations used for comparison were the candidates' actual NCLEX-RN results from the July 1990 or February 1991 administrations.

Operational data on CAT administration were obtained using several types of test administration centers for the CAT field testing. The CAT field testing was conducted in commercial testing centers, a community college computer laboratory, university computer laboratories, and state computer training laboratories. Logistical information and additional stakeholder buy-in was also obtained by field testing CAT in eight states with diverse characteristics (California, Illinois, Mississippi, Missouri, New Jersey, New York, Oregon, and Texas). Candidates also provided information about their CAT experience via a post-examination questionnaire.

Results of the psychometric comparisons of the July 1990 and February 1991 CAT field test and the paper-and-pencil versions of the NCLEX were generally positive and suggested that CAT examinations could produce comparable results to the paper-and-pencil NCLEX.[8] The operational data were also very positive regarding CAT feasibility. State personnel were trained successfully to conduct the CAT administration and each state administered the CAT field testing without major difficulty. The different CAT administration environments were not a major factor in candidate performance. Candidate satisfaction with the settings for CAT administration was fairly consistent, although the college laboratories were rated slightly lower in quality control compared to the professional testing centers. On average, candidates spent approximately the same time on each CAT question as was allocated during the paper-and-pencil NCLEX administration. The field tests uncovered no psychometric or operational impediments to proceeding with the project.

The CAT legal analysis was conducted by the University of Illinois Office of Social Science Research and the legal firm of Vedder, Price, Kaufman & Kammholz. Two lines of legal analysis were initiated: a psychometric and legal literature review, and legal opinion as briefs. The legal briefs addressed three features that make CAT different operationally than standard paper-and-pencil licensure testing: (1) the computerized nature of the test, (2) the adaptive nature of the test, and (3) the CAT examination stopping rules. The preliminary CAT legal analysis found wide-ranging support for using CAT as a testing methodology. The researchers found no direct case law addressing CAT and few cases on important psychometric issues surrounding CAT. The University of Illinois researchers concluded that there are no obvious legal impediments to implementing CAT for licensure, given the proper psychometric evidence for the validity of the CAT version of the examination.

Vedder, Price, Kaufman & Kammholz conducted a more detailed legal analysis. This detailed analysis developed a list of issues surrounding CAT with substantive legal conclusions, developed a list of key issues requiring psychometric evidence, and identified issues that assisted in the design of the CAT examination process. The legal opinion briefs together suggested that if the psychometric properties of the CAT are sound, and candidates are notified about the CAT procedures prior to testing, then there should be no obvious legal impediments to implementing CAT as one of the steps in the nurse licensure process.

The entire legal analysis was published as a separate monograph, *Collected Works on the Legal Aspects of Computerized Adaptive Testing[9]*. On the basis of the psychometric, operational, security, and legal information provided during the course of Phases I and II, the Delegate Assembly decided to implement CAT for administering the NCLEX. Their second decision was to develop a request for proposals (RFP) to secure bids for providing computerized testing services.

Decisions during the request for proposal and vendor selection process. The development of the request for proposal (RFP) for testing services and the vendor selection process offered an important opportunity to shape the direction of the operational CAT program. The National Council's RFP defined the major service areas in four categories: (1) test development and research, (2) data services, (3) test administration, and (4) a national Beta Test in which all boards of nursing were encouraged to participate. The Beta Test was an important part of the RFP and it provided boards of nursing with one final opportunity to obtain CAT performance information for NCLEX before beginning the operational program. National Council decided to require the conduct of a Beta Test based on a number of informational needs:

1. The determination of whether the paper-and-pencil NCLEX passing standard would translate as equivalent to CAT administration of NCLEX.
2. A live test of the computer data transfer systems.
3. A tryout of operational board processes.
4. The desire to actually try out the nationwide test center network.

Along with the features of the proposed test development and research, data services, administration, and cost, the quality of the Beta Test designed by the testing service vendors also was important in the vendor selection by the Delegate Assembly.

Decisions about the final implementation date. Due to the timing of the National Council's annual Delegate Assembly meetings and the desire to implement CAT as soon as it was ready, the final implementation timeline decision ("readiness decision") was assigned to the National Council's Board of Directors. The Delegate Assembly approved the readiness criteria, but the decision about when to implement was given to the Board. The Beta Test was designed to provide results which would inform the Board of Directors about the operational readiness of the entire CAT system for administering NCLEX. The Board was responsible for developing the final implementation timeline after evaluating the results of the Beta Test (see Way[10] for a discussion of the Beta Test results). The concept of "readiness" to proceed with the CAT implementation was defined on the basis of Beta Test results, preparation by boards of nursing, and the vendor test service's preparation. The key issues were:

1. Psychometrics (candidate and item analyses, passing standard transfer).
2. Item pools (size, quality).
3. Security (items, candidate information).
4. Sites (at least one in each state, equipment, staff training).
5. Site and board system procedures (eligibility notices, proctoring, results reporting).
6. Data transfer (sites to test services, boards to test services, test services to boards).
7. Communications (to candidates, educators, boards).

As discussed previously, the National Council played a significant role in assisting boards of nursing to prepare for CAT administration of NCLEX. The Board of Directors' implementation timeline decision was complicated by the Delegate Assembly's determination that the transition to CAT would occur at a single point in time for all boards. That is, after conversion, paper-and-pencil versions of NCLEX would not be offered. This one-time implementation process meant that a significant majority of boards of nursing needed to be able to legally and operationally administer NCLEX using CAT prior to setting the final timeline. This caused National Council to closely monitor the operational Beta Test results and also work with boards of nursing which needed legislation or rule changes to enable CAT administration of NCLEX.

National Council's CAT Implementation Timeline

As with most efforts in a new project, at the start of Phase I, the National Council had not defined all the steps or processes for conversion into a coherent whole. Thus, the project timeline may have stretched longer than what could be optimally accomplished by an organization with a different decision-making structure or a different tolerance for risk. Figure 1 illustrates a successful conversion timeline and it shows only the National Council's major transition steps in going from a paper-and-pencil to a CAT implementation of the national nurse licensure examination, NCLEX:

Figure 1

<table>
<tr><td colspan="2" align="center">**Timeline for Conversion of NCLEX to CAT**</td></tr>
<tr><td>1986 December</td><td>Appoint Project Committee</td></tr>
<tr><td>1987 February</td><td>Hire Project Director, Begin Phase I</td></tr>
<tr><td>1988 August</td><td>Report Phase I Outcomes, Delegate Assembly Authorized Phase II</td></tr>
<tr><td>1990 July</td><td>Field Test RNs</td></tr>
<tr><td>1991 February</td><td>Field Test RNs</td></tr>
<tr><td>1991 August</td><td>Report Phase II Outcomes; Delegate Assembly Decision to Approve CAT for NCLEX</td></tr>
<tr><td>1991 September</td><td>Request for Proposals (RFP) Issued to Potential NCLEX/CAT Test Service Vendors</td></tr>
<tr><td>1992 January</td><td>CAT Test Service Proposals Received; Begin Evaluation and Negotiation</td></tr>
<tr><td>1992 August</td><td>Delegate Assembly Selected ETS and SLS as Contractors for CAT Testing Services</td></tr>
<tr><td>1992 October</td><td>Field Test PNs; Began Major Preparation for the NCLEX Beta Test of the National CAT Measurement System for NCLEX</td></tr>
<tr><td>1993 April</td><td>Communicated About Beta Testing at National Council's Regional Meetings</td></tr>
<tr><td>1993 June-July</td><td>Conducted NCLEX Beta Test</td></tr>
<tr><td>1993 August</td><td>Delegate Assembly Approved the Decision Criteria for Determining the Actual Timing of CAT Implementation (Readiness Criteria)</td></tr>
<tr><td>1993 October</td><td>Board of Directors' Decision on CAT Systematic Readiness</td></tr>
<tr><td>1994 April 1</td><td>Nationally Implement CAT for NCLEX</td></tr>
<tr><td>1996 August</td><td>Conduct Evaluation of NCLEX</td></tr>
</table>

Conclusions

The conversion to CAT implemented by the National Council required significant effort and commitment of organizational resources. Early work included a review of the psychometric requirements of CAT, an assessment of how close the NCLEX was to meeting the requirements, and a plan to provide for the needed but not-yet attained requirements. Much planning was devoted to the organizational decision-making process and development of materials and information which facilitated those decisions. During the study of CAT feasibility for NCLEX, critical issues were investigated and addressed concerning psychometrics, legal defensibility, operational processes, and security. Identification of all stakeholders and their interests was an integral part of the conversion, both from the perspective of providing quality service to boards of nursing and from a candidate fairness perspective. The process for selecting testing services and test administration vendors provided an opportunity to assess the state-of-the-art in CAT administration and fine-tune the contract requirements to encompass all of the important test development, administration, security, and reporting needs.

The technical and psychometric challenges in moving an existing high-stakes, paper-and-pencil testing program to CAT administration are formidable. Even beyond the technical challenges, the necessary groundwork cannot be overlooked in bringing all the stakeholders along throughout the decision-making and planning process. In fact, these "softer" work efforts take as much time and resources as setting up the technical capabilities to actually conduct national CAT examinations. The successful transition from a familiar paper-and-pencil testing modality to an unfamiliar and new CAT modality is dependent on attending to countless psychometric, operational, systems, personnel, educational, and communications details.

References

1. Hambleton RK, Swaminathan H. *Item Response Theory: Principles and Applications*. Boston: Kluwer-Nihoff Publishing, 1985.

2. Rasch G. *Probabilistic models for some intelligence and attainment tests*. Copenhagen: Danmarks Paedagogiske Institut, 1960.

3. Hofer PJ, Green BF The challenge of competence and creativity in computerized psychological testing. *Consult Clin Psychol*, 1985; 53: 826-838.

4. Kiely GL, Zara AR, Weiss DJ. *Equivalence of computer-administered and paper-and-pencil ASVAB tests* (AFHRL-TP-86-13). Manpower and Personnel Division, Brooks Air Force Base, TX: Air Force Human Resources Laboratory, 1986.

5. National Council of State Boards of Nursing. *Model Nursing Practice Act.* Chicago: National Council of State Boards of Nursing, August, 1988a.

6. National Council of State Boards of Nursing. *Model Nursing Administrative Rules.* Chicago: National Council of State Boards of Nursing. August 1988b.

7. Kingsbury GG, Zara AR. Procedures for selecting items for computerized adaptive tests. *Appl Meas Educ,* 1989; 2:359-375.

8. Zara AR. A comparison of computerized adaptive and paper-and-pencil versions of the national RN licensure examination. Paper presented at the Annual Meeting of the *American Educational Research Association,* San Francisco, April 1992.

9. National Council of State Boards of Nursing. *Collected Works on the Legal Aspects of Computerized Adaptive Testing.* Chicago. National Council of State Boards of Nursing, 1985.

10. Way WD. Psychometric results of the NCLEX™ Beta Test. Paper presented at the Annual Meeting of the *American Educational Research Association,* New Orleans, March 1994.

Certifying Boards and Computer-Based Examinations

William H. Hartmann, M.D.
American Board of Pathology

The American Board of Pathology (Abpath) gave its first certification examinations to 60 physician pathologists in May 1936, and has administered certification examinations throughout the intervening 60 years. Of the Member Boards of the American Board of Medical Specialties (ABMS) the ABPath is one that entirely controls its examination process. There are, presently, 15 test committees (comprising pathologists who are experts in the field) meeting regularly to create, review, and accept questions for future examinations. The test committees also review and comment on the examination grids ("test blueprints") which serve as the scaffold on which trustees create the certifying examinations.

Accepted questions are reviewed by ABPath staff for style, grammar, and spelling, and are entered into the test item bank. At present, the item bank contains about 25,000 items composed of 18,000 written questions, 5,000 questions with illustrations, and 2,000 questions with glass slides for the microscopic examinations. Test items are selected by the trustees from the item bank and the ABPath staff construct the examinations. Examinations are administered by the ABPath trustees and staff, usually twice a year, at preselected sites around the country. The examination answer sheets are scored; performance statistics are created for each item, and outliers are reviewed for rejection by the responsible trustee. Examination statistics are created following review by a committee of trustees, and pass/fail letters sent to each candidate. All items are returned to the data bank, outlier items being referred to the responsible test committee for review and decision as to whether to continue to include the question. The ABPath's psychometrician prepares a written report on the performance of each examination compared to previous administrations, and comments on items of interest.

91

In the early 1960s John J. Andujar, M.D., then a trustee of the ABPath, started the ABPath on the road to computerization. He campaigned aggressively, as reflected in the board minutes, to convince his fellow trustees of the need to move to an automated scoring system. He convinced them to begin to use IBM "Port-a-Punch" cards and optically scannable answer sheets during the examination (for candidates), and by the trustees in place of the laborious manual scoring of the examinations the evening after an administration. This automated scoring system finally was adopted in 1967 for most, if not all, examinations.

Under the guidance of Murray R. Abell, M.D., Ph.D., Executive Vice President, of the ABPath, computerization continued through the years for office preparation and examination scoring. No formal process for computer-based examination administration appeared, however, until 1993.

In February 1993 representatives of the American Boards of Family Practice, Internal Medicine, Orthopaedic Surgery, and the ABMS were invited to the ABPath for a one day meeting to share experience about the use of computers and computer systems for certification examinations. The trustees of the ABPath had previously decided to proceed with the creation of a process to update handling of office data and to explore using a computer system for the certification examinations. These trustee actions led to the relocation of the ABPath office and to building an examination facility as part of the new office. The examination facility contains 46 computer workstations, each having a dedicated computer, monitor, mouse, and keyboard situated on an L-shaped desk (Figure 1). One side of the L will be used for a microscope when such is an integral part of an examination. Computer requirements for each station are listed in Figure 2.

Figure 1

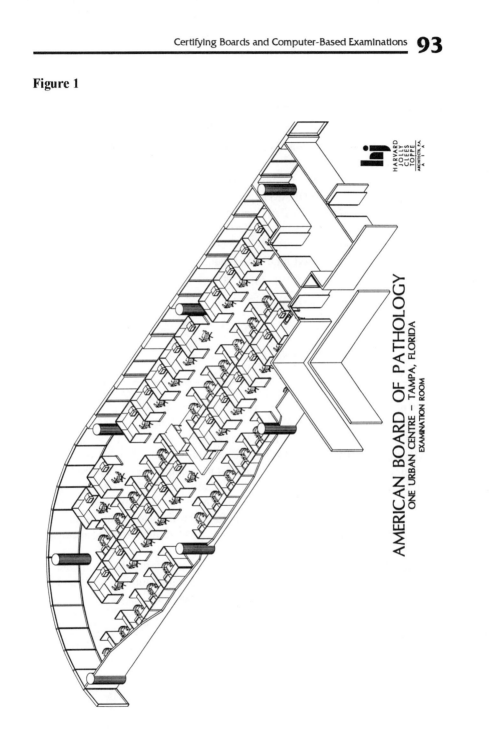

AMERICAN BOARD OF PATHOLOGY
ONE URBAN CENTRE – TAMPA, FLORIDA
EXAMINATION ROOM

HARVARD
JOLLY
CLEES
TOPPE
ARCHITECTS, P.A.
A I A

Figure 2

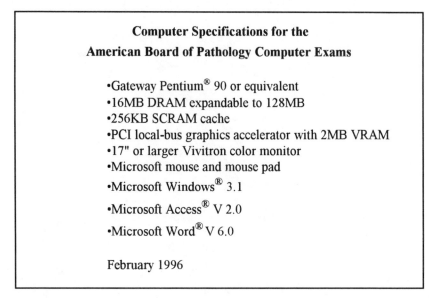

**Computer Specifications for the
American Board of Pathology Computer Exams**

•Gateway Pentium® 90 or equivalent
•16MB DRAM expandable to 128MB
•256KB SCRAM cache
•PCI local-bus graphics accelerator with 2MB VRAM
•17" or larger Vivitron color monitor
•Microsoft mouse and mouse pad
•Microsoft Windows® 3.1
•Microsoft Access® V 2.0
•Microsoft Word® V 6.0

February 1996

There is a raised proctors area in the center of the room and an adjacent registration area. Both the registration area and the workstation area have their own entrances off of a main corridor. The examination room is 1,775 square feet. The hardware, software, and furniture cost approximately $400,000.

With the help of a consultant, a request-for-proposal (RFP) was developed in April 1993. Mrs. Beth Hammond of the ABPath's staff was given authority for program development. An additional consultant (Dr. Richard Rovinelli) was recruited. In October 1994 a vendor conference was held in the examination room-to-be. Proposals were due in November 1994. Contracts were awarded in January 1995.

On 17 July 1995 twenty-four candidates for certification in blood banking/transfusion medicine were examined, via the ABPath computer system. There were no untoward events (Figure 3). We were successful!!!

Figure 3

The First ABPath Computer-Based Examination

July 17, 1995

Blood Banking on a computer!
What a way to take an exam!

Twenty some candidates filed into the room,
Twenty some testees first time at the "Board."
The silence was awesome
but twas the "noise" of success.

No real problems apparent to me.
We'll have to wait and see
what comments we get from
the twenty some testees.

First run of workbooks for the written.
One candidate was really smitten,
for on his book he wrote a great deal
of how the system we could change
to make it more real.

Move a button from here to there.
Label them all so that even the
weak or timid could sense those
that were really meant to be.

Even test items in writing he corrected.
Perhaps he had not enough
to do while taking the exam?

Others commented not at all
but used the pages for
scribbling as a child would upon a wall.

And so it came and went
this day of days this
most significant certification event.
Not with a shout or a hosanna
but with a smile of satisfaction
that we had turned a pathway
towards a nirvana.

William H. Hartmann, M.D.
17 July 1995

In August and September of 1995 certification examinations also were administered in chemical pathology and medical microbiology. The same computer-based examination system was used, and again the process was successful. The ABPath had accomplished what it set out to do: successfully administer certification examinations via a computer system.

The examinations represent the use of a computer system to administer the examination. The computer replaces the examination books. There has been little change in examination format (ABPath uses multiple-choice questions), but some modification became necessary either because of computer screen size limitations, digitization of test questions, or examination room configuration. Each problem was solved in an acceptable and appropriate way with full support of the ABPath trustees. The psychometric analysis of these multiple-choice examinations revealed no performance differences from previous examinations in these specialties.

As the candidates left an examination they were asked to complete a short questionnaire and all but one did so. The results seem to confirm our opinion of the success (Figure 4).

Figure 4

Candidates' Comments on
Computer-Based Examinations in 1995

1) How comfortable are you using a computer?

NOT AT ALL	COMFORTABLE	VERY COMFORTABLE
3	14	24

2) Have you previously taken an examination on a computer?

No	ONCE OR TWICE	MANY TIMES
36	2	3

3) Were The American Board of Pathology instructions clear?

No	MORE OR LESS	VERY
	9	32

4) How was the quality of the images? (Applies to one examination)

NOT ACCEPTABLE	ACCEPTABLE	EXCELLENT
10	1	1

5) Were the examination facilities comfortable?

No	MORE OR LESS	VERY COMFORTABLE
	11	30

6) Do you think the length of time allowed for the examination appropriate?

No	MORE OR LESS	YES
3	6	32

We were also successful in the eyes of the candidates. The ABPath expects to administer three subspecialty examinations in 1996 using this system. Two of these examinations will represent a new format. Both will use microscopes as part of the testing process. In 1997, eight examinations are expected to be computer-based. The ABPath has begun to explore how a similar system could be used for other ABPath certifying examinations which, at present, have many more candidates than can be accommodated in the 46 module examination facility.

The ABPath has no magical solutions to offer anyone who may be considering such a change. Computerization of certifying examinations is a problem to be solved and should be approached the same way individual organizations approach and solve other problems. Success for ABPath rests clearly on the shoulders of those who had the vision to proceed: Dr. Andujar, Dr. Abell, Mrs. Hammond, Dr. Rovinelli, and the trustees of the American Board of Pathology.

Candidates and Computer-Based Examinations

Fred G. Smith, M.D.
American Board of Pediatrics

The American Board of Pediatrics (ABPeds) began administering a voluntary, open-book, written recertification examination in 1980; however, very few diplomates participated in this program. In 1985, the ABPeds began to reassess the recertification process and concluded that the methodology of recertification would have to be changed. It was decided that one of the major goals of recertification would be to stimulate life-long learning and thereby maintain an acceptable level of clinical knowledge throughout the practice years. As a result of its deliberations, the ABPeds decided in 1988 to begin issuing time-limited, seven-year certificates. The voluntary proctored written recertification examination process ended in 1992.

The ABPeds desired to develop a recertification process that would test not only cognitive knowledge but also other competencies such as the ability to work through diagnostic problems and their management. It became apparent that it would be difficult to have several written examination components, give the examination at home, and still have some degree of security. The ABPeds, therefore, explored the use of computers to administer an examination that would test knowledge, diagnostic ability, and management of patients. It was decided that a computer-based examination would be developed that was open-book, given at home or other convenient location, was user-friendly, and was as secure as possible. The security of the examination would be enhanced by randomizing questions in the same examination, frequently changing examination content, using a computerized test item selection, encrypting the examination material, and employing a timer which causes data to "self-destruct" after a set date.

Once the decision was made to have a three-component (Knowledge, Diagnosis, and Management), computer-based examination, the board recruited programmers and program analysts to develop the software to administer the examination components. In 1988, when development started, the software to assist in the examination development was scarce and the programming languages to formulate the programs were difficult and cumbersome to use compared with the sophisticated hardware and graphic user interface software available today. The three components included: *Knowledge* testing, using multiple-choice questions; *Diagnosis*, in which the candidate starts out with a vignette describing the presenting complaint, works through the process of taking a medical history, a physical examination, and selecting appropriate laboratory studies, and then makes a diagnosis; and *Management* which begins with a history, physical examination, and laboratory studies to allow the candidate to make a diagnosis and proceed with the management of a patient.

Help Desk and Participant Surveys

Since the inception of the Program for Renewal of Certification in Pediatrics - Computer (PRCP-C), information regarding the participants' concerns and issues has been collected by the ABPeds help desk. Assistance from the help desk is available during the day and at night, seven days a week, and provides assistance with any technical problems the participant may be confronted with. Information is also collected through a questionnaire at the end of the computer examination components. The ABPeds also encourages comments from participants regarding their concerns about examination content and, thus far, this has resulted in many letters and phone calls, some with references to support their concerns. These comments are utilized in the question validation process. The ABPeds underestimated the number of comments and critiques to be received regarding the content of the examinations and had to develop a method to respond to these. The ABPeds felt that even though it was time consuming to respond, it did have a positive side in that it reinforced the ABPeds' impression that the participants spend a great deal of time researching the answers to the questions in the examination components.

Participant Issues and Concerns

Because a computer is needed to take the examination, and there are three different examinations on computer diskettes, the ABPeds anticipated that some significant participant concerns would have to be addressed.

Figure 1

Issues and Concerns of Participants

•Computer literacy
•Access to a computer
•Time commitment
•Cost
•Content

Taking the Examination on a Computer

Thirty percent of the participants at the start of PRCP-C did not have access to a computer, and many of those who had access expressed fear of using a computer to take an examination. The problems encountered in completing the computer-based examination seemed to reflect their limited knowledge about computers. There were many general inquiries about simple tasks such as installing and de-installing exam diskettes, forgetting to turn on the monitor, or not properly inserting the diskettes into the drive. The ABPeds anticipated these general and technical inquiries and developed several strategies to address their concerns and alleviate their fears. These included: the establishment of a help desk for technical problems; hands-on demonstrations at national meetings of the American Academy of Pediatrics (AAP); special continuing medical education courses conducted by the AAP; and user-friendly tutorials at the beginning of each examination component. In addition, the examination software was designed to operate using only a few keys on the computer keyboard, other keys remaining inoperative. There was a dramatic decrease in the total number of calls per examination component shipped after the initial few months.

Access to a Computer

Accessibility to a computer was a concern of both the candidates and the ABPeds. The ABPeds felt this issue would be short-term (four to five years) because medical students and residents presently in training programs were becoming much more computer literate, since computers are used more frequently in office management, education, and to gather information. Prior to initiating PRCP-C, based on a random survey of diplomates of ABPeds in 1991, approximately 70 percent had immediate access either to an IBM-compatible or Macintosh® personal computer. Follow-up surveys suggest that over 85 percent of the PRCP-C participants take the examination at home; the remainder use an office computer. The Macintosh® users currently must use emulation software to run the IBM-compatible PRCP-C software. The ABPeds recognizes this as a significant participant problem. At the end of 1996, however, both Macintosh® and Windows® versions will be available. The ABPeds postponed development of a Macintosh® version because of the significant additional cost, and the availability of emulation software for the Macintosh®. With the availability today of new software allowing cross-platform development at minimal added cost, the ABPeds would have developed programs for Macintosh® and Windows® as well as DOS. (DOS is the common computer "diskette operating system.")

Time Commitment

During the initial three months, nearly all of the participants started with the *Knowledge* component (a 300 multiple-choice question examination). Even though the pilot-testing suggested that 300 questions was a reasonable number, the candidates complained that it took 15-20 hours or more to complete the test, and a significant percentage (15 percent) were spending over 25 hours.

Since the people pilot testing the examinations were not taking the examination for recertification purposes, the disparity between the pilot testers and the participants was attributed to the participants' concern about passing the examinations. Comments and verbal feedback also confirmed the impression that they were consulting references to verify their answers. At the end of each examination component, a survey now asks about the amount of time the participant took to complete the examination, what educational resources (e.g., textbooks, journals, CME courses) were used to prepare, and what resources were used during the examination.

Figure 2

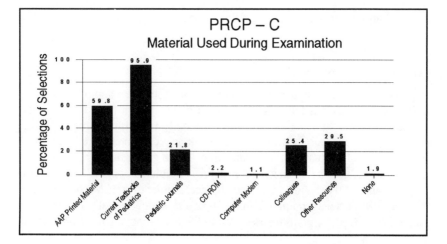

The American Academy of Pediatrics (AAP) developed an educational program, Pediatrics Review and Education Program (PREP), to assist pediatricians in preparing for recertification. PREP also includes a computer-based self-assessment examination. As illustrated in Figure 2, a majority of the PRCP participants use both current pediatric textbooks and the PREP, but many use other resources, too. Even when the number of required questions was reduced to 120, participants still took an average of 11-12 hours to complete the *Knowledge* component. About the same time is required to complete the other two components, *Diagnosis* and *Management.*

Figure 3

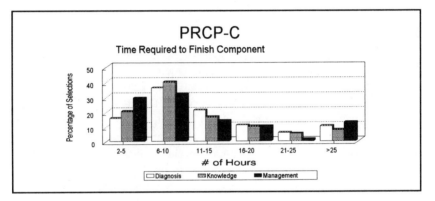

Cost of the Examination

Cost was a major concern not only of the candidates, but also of the ABPeds. Costs were underestimated for developing a complex, comprehensive, open-book, at-home, computer-based examination. At the time development started, limited technology and computer software was available to develop and administer computer-based examinations. Programming was more cumbersome and time consuming. Development costs were in excess of $1.5 million per year during the first three years. Coupled with a relatively small number of diplomates who had to be recertified each year, the development costs contributed to the necessity for a relatively high examination fee. If more diplomates with unlimited time certificates took the examination, the cost would be significantly less.

Participants continue to comment on the high cost of certificate fees even though the ABPeds has pointed out that the examinations can be taken at home, thereby eliminating the expense of travel to an examination site and lost income because of being away from their practice. Fee increases have been below the consumer price index, and it is anticipated that the fee may be further modified downward when diplomates with time-limited certificates begin recertifying again around the turn of the century.

Content of the Examination

Unlike a proctored written examination, participants taking the computer-based examination have the opportunity to research each question or problem and to send comments and critiques when they return their examination diskettes. The ABPeds encourages these comments about content. Thus far, this encouragement has resulted in many letters and phone calls, some with references to support their concerns. The comments are used in the test question validation process. The ABPeds underestimated the number of comments and critiques regarding examination content, and had to develop a method to respond. Even though it was time consuming to respond, there is a positive side; it reinforced one goal of the PRCP-C: continuing medical education.

Summary

The ABPeds responded to the participants' concerns and issues in a timely fashion and as problems arose with examination software, corrections were made so that the examination components have become very user friendly from both the participants' and the board's viewpoints. During the past six months, most participants' concerns are about test content, the need to use emulation software for Macintosh® computers, and the examination fee. The ABPeds worked closely with the AAP, as the AAP developed and offers their Pediatrics Review and Education Program (PREP) based on the ABPeds' examination content specifications. The AAP leadership also has emphasized the need for recertification, and has been supportive of PRCP.

In addition, the hardware available to participants at home or in the office must be considered, for example, the introduction of graphics in the examination may require more sophisticated equipment than most participants may have available.

Figure 4

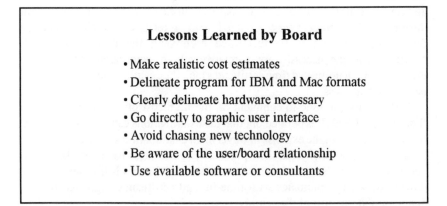

Lessons Learned by Board

- Make realistic cost estimates
- Delineate program for IBM and Mac formats
- Clearly delineate hardware necessary
- Go directly to graphic user interface
- Avoid chasing new technology
- Be aware of the user/board relationship
- Use available software or consultants

Discussion

Charles P. Friedman, Ph.D. (University of North Carolina): Dr. Smith, I was interested in your comments about the cross-platform issues, especially if you are dealing with examinees who are taking the exam at home. There is a lot of mythology about how many Macintosh® computers (Macs) really exist. A lot of people who use personal computers (PCs) in the office are said to have a Macintosh® at home. Do you know how many of your examinees actually took their exam on Macs and whether there is a trend?

Fred G. Smith, M.D. (American Board of Pediatrics): Originally about 10-12 percent of generalists used Macs in a survey we made before we started, and it looks like it still would be about 10 percent Mac® users now. About that time software for PCs came along and we decided that instead of spending $300,000 to $400,000 to develop software for the Mac, we would go with the newer PC software. That may have been a bad decision. About 22 to 25 percent of subspecialists have Macintosh® computers, and they are a very vocal group. They love their Macs and I think we made a mistake.

Paul Martin (American Board of Otolaryngology): I have several questions. When you are using computerized tests, have you given any thought to the idea of somebody printing the contents of the screen (the actual question and answer on a printer)? What are the security measures for that? What about writing down questions and answers? What precludes a candidate from copying a test when it is taken at home? I know there is an honor system, but is there more? I also feel somebody will complain that they are discriminated against because they cannot use a computer properly. Is there a need for a written test for people who do not use computers? Does anyone on the panel have a policy or plan on this issue?

Dr. Smith: The issue of computer literacy was a very major problem for us. A very small minority of people, again very vocal, felt discriminated against. We finally developed a written exam; it is given at five sites once a year to a small percentage of pediatricians. So far two examinations have been or will be administered; one last year for 113 diplomates and one in April with 83 registered so far.

Anthony R. Zara, Ph.D. (National Council of State Boards of Nursing): For the National Council examination, because it is given at professional test sites, the "print screen" keyboard option is inactivated, and tests are given at professional work stations. We do not worry about candidates printing questions. Just as for the paper-and-pencil test, we give them scratch paper which is counted before the test and after the test. We have not run across a specific "life" problem that does not allow a person to use a computer. For test accommodations we allow pretty much the same as for paper-and-pencil tests; if a reader, a recorder, or a separate room is needed, we can provide that in a computer-based test.

William H. Hartmann, M.D. (American Board of Pathology): We are moving ahead with the at-home recertification examination which will be given again at the end of this year. Basically, we view questions on the at-home examination as lost. Once the disks leave the office, for practical purposes test questions are not available to use again. We also follow the same procedure Dr. Zara described, namely deactivate "print screen" key in examinations at home or tests in the office. In the examination center that I demonstrated to you, candidates are not given any paper. We have not had to confront the issue of the totally "computer-shy" candidate at the present time. My guess is that we would probably treat the situation in the same way that we treat any extraordinary request for an examination.

Ivan Damjanov, M.D. (University of Kansas Medical Center): The question is for Dr. Zara. In my medical school I noted a flurry of new test review companies who cater to nurses. I am impressed with the sophistication that they use in marketing and selling diskettes. You probably know of these companies. How much piracy is there? How much do they try to infiltrate the boards? How much cross pollination is there? How do you deal with these companies? Do you have any contact with them?

Dr. Zara: Yes, these companies are an ongoing concern. I am not sure that the move to computer-based testing has made the problem different. The licensure boards in nursing have had procedures in place to assure that the candidates who come to take the paper examination are known. Those security measures have been duplicated for computer testing. In terms of security at the site, we implemented a digitized photograph. Every candidate, before he or she takes the exam, must sit and get a photograph; it is attached to their results report and follows them throughout their career. We think the digital photograph has gone a long way to stop fraudulent taking of exams.

Protecting test items from review courses again uses the standard security agreements in terms of copyrighting items and having candidates sign an agreement that they will not misuse the test questions. Both steps help protect us *after* the fact. If candidates memorize questions and take them out of the room, we are protected somewhat, because the boards approve candidate eligibility. Only real candidates can sit for examinations and not people that work for the review companies. The test is computer adaptive and I think memorizing any small subset of questions really does not help. If someone fails and has memorized questions from the last time, they will not see those questions again. The way tailored testing works is, if they answer questions correctly that their ability would not normally allow them to answer correctly, the test presents questions their ability level cannot support and they will get those questions wrong, falling down to the lower ability level. We feel confident with these security measures.

In terms of cultivating relationships with the test review companies, again that is a double-edged sword. We try to mail the companies our internal publications, and our newsletters. We have a quarterly publication sent to them that discusses Council research and Council projects. It really does help if they have the correct information and we try our best to make sure we answer all their questions.

Dr. Hartmann: There is one other aspect of this whole business which has not come up and I do not think it will come up later; i.e., the issue of examination copyright. The American Board of Pathology has copyrighted all of its examinations for many, many years. We have just begun to deal with the copyright office with reference to copyrighting the computer-based examinations. It is much more difficult. You need to be sensitive to that problem. A copyright infringement could go a long way to preclude future use of the examination. Copyrighting computer-based tests can be done, but it is not easy.

LESSONS LEARNED ABOUT SIMULATIONS

PART

5

The Experience of the
National Board of Medical Examiners*
(or "Success Seems Always Just Over the Horizon")

Donald E. Melnick, M.D.
National Board of Medical Examiners

When asked, almost a year ago, if I would speak about the National Board's experience with computer-based examinations, I had somewhat mixed feelings. On the one hand, it has been a tremendous personal privilege to be connected with the National Board of Medical Examiners' (NBME) efforts to exploit computer technology to improve testing. On the other hand, it is a little bit embarrassing to describe a nearly 30-year old project to develop the centerpiece tool, computer-based case simulations, for the National Board's computer-based testing plans. I feel a bit like Tom Hanks' character in the movie *Big*, having spent the last 13 years playing with computers. But, after 30 years of contribution by eminent leaders in American medicine, not to mention the largest chunk of my professional career, where is the product? As Alexander Pope said, "Hope springs eternal in the human breast." So I have subtitled this presentation "Success seems always just over the horizon."

The voyage, from research panel recommendations in 1968 to plans to use computer-based testing in the United States Medical Licensing Examination (USMLE) in the imminent future, has navigated stormy seas. As a prelude to reviewing my personal perspectives of the key issues and key lessons learned on this voyage, I want to highlight some major stages of the journey (Figure 1).

*© National Board of Medical Examiners, 1996

111

Figure 1

NBME Voyage of Discovery with Computer-Based Testing

1968-1970 *NBME Research Advisory Committee*
  - Recommends NBME develop computer-based system to test physician skills previously tested in bedside examinations.

1970-1975 *Exploring Simulations*
  - Developed diagnostic and physiologic models.
  - Explored Bayesian scoring.
  - Developed computerized patient management problems (PMPs).

1975-1982 *The Patient Management Model*
  - Developed management paradigm for simulation model that is uncued, time realistic and includes scoring system.

1983-1989 *Case Development and Personal Computers*
  - Moved to personal computer platform, added audio/video.
  - Developed methods to mass produce cases.
  - Item response theory (IRT) scoring model explored.
  - Developed multiple-choice question systems for computer.
  - 1988 field trials undertaken.
  - CTL Inc. created/abandoned for delivery of computerized examinations.

1990-1994 *Scoring and Dissemination*
  - Distributed simulation systems to medical schools.
  - Developed expert-based scoring systems.
  - Refined case development technology.
  - Developed graphical display system.

1995-1999 *Implementation*
  - USMLE strategic plan adopted: convert USMLE Step 1 and Step 2 exams to computer administration, use case simulations in Step 3.
  - Selected commercial vendor for test delivery.
  - Converted Special Purpose Examination (SPEX) to computer.

The impetus for the National Board's efforts to apply computer technology to assessment programs was clearly linked to the decision made by the Board in the early 1960s to eliminate the bedside clinical component from its Part III examination. It was with great reluctance that the National Board bowed to the mounting evidence that these exams were unfair. Examinations lacking tools to more directly assess clinical skills than was possible with multiple-choice question (MCQ) tests have never been fully acceptable to the National Board's leadership.

In 1968 the National Board's Research Advisory Committee (Alexander Barry, Robert Ebel, T. Hale Ham, William Mayer, Jack Myers, Kenneth Rogers, Dael Wolfle, and Louis Welt) recommended that the National Board develop a computer-based simulation system to test the physician skills previously tested in bedside examinations. A prototype simulation of an initial patient diagnostic model was demonstrated at the American College of Physicians' meeting in 1970.

From 1970-1975 work continued as a joint effort with the American Board of Internal Medicine (ABIM). During this phase five models were developed and/or evaluated. The INDEX system allowed the physician to obtain history, physical examination, and some test results by entering numbers from a coded list. After ten minutes the physician had to provide a diagnosis. The CASE system functioned much like INDEX but exploited a free-text input for the questions asked by the physician. MATRIX required the physician to make a diagnosis based on cues and used Bayesian probability to score the accuracy of the diagnostic decisions. The computerized PMP was a traditional patient management problem without the disadvantage of backtracking. CRISYS was a physiologic cardiovascular simulator with dynamic patient response to interventions. Each model was tested and student and physician reactions collected and evaluated.

From 1975 to 1982 the joint NBME/ABIM project continued at the University of Wisconsin. The focus of effort during this phase was the development of a management model which realistically avoided cueing and simulated the movement of time. Patient care, as in real life, no longer ended with the diagnosis but required continued management of the patient. The first bona fide scoring systems were developed based on PMP work, and a large field trial was conducted.

During the next phase the National Board and ABIM parted ways. NBME continued to work independently on the project. A study by the Yankee Group and subsequent consultation with Boeing Computer Services led to the conclusion that the simulation system should be reprogrammed for the then new personal computer. In fact, the first Delaware Valley 80286 machines were obtained for this project through the efforts of Boeing Computer Services, since previous machines could not meet the memory requirements of the model as it was being programmed. The model was enriched by the addition of images and sound delivered using interactive analogue video disks. Ground-breaking work with AT&T Bell Laboratories developed some of the key technologies for digital enhancement of medical images to support the NBME effort.

In earlier phases, cases had been laboriously hand crafted by individual clinicians and uniquely programmed. We developed mass production technologies for cases using the familiar committee structure of the NBME. We were able to produce approximately 200 cases over a three-year period. We refined scoring models by applying an item-response theory-based, partial credit analytic model that allowed us to handle scoring-related actions on a continuum of correctness and to accommodate for different pathways taken through the same case by different examinees.

Recognizing that computer administration of simulated cases would make paper-and-pencil administration of MCQs appear outmoded, we also developed systems to support computer administration of multiple-choice question tests. Major effort was expended at the NBME to prepare the Part III examinations for computer administration. Extensive field trials of the new systems, cases, and the MCQ test were conducted in 1987-1988. An advisory panel concluded from these results that "CBX succeeded in measuring a quality not measured by MCQ and PMP tests that may reasonably be considered to be related to general clinical competence." The results of these trials were presented in an invitational conference sponsored by the NBME in March 1988.

Concurrently with this work, the NBME was attempting to create an infrastructure that would allow computer delivery of its examinations. In 1986 it created CTL, Inc. as a wholly-owned subsidiary for this purpose. I have a rare first and only edition of CTL's marketing brochure entitled "The First Nationwide Network of CBT Interactive Video Centers." In 1988, recognizing that the initial business plan for CTL was overly optimistic, the NBME withdrew its support and the subsidiary was closed. Clearly an idea that was ahead of its time, CTL worked with several clients who subsequently found other outlets for computer-based testing, including the National Council of State Boards of Nursing and the National Council of Architectural Review Boards (NCARB). Both now have active computer-based testing programs. The National Council program was described this morning and the NCARB program is now in a pilot testing phase of an architectural simulation.

Primarily because of the lack of a delivery vehicle but also because of refinements needed in case scoring, the planned 1989 implementation of case simulations in Part III was indefinitely deferred. Since 1989 development work has continued unabated. Now the project focused on dissemination of the case simulation technology to medical schools. More than 90 medical schools in the U.S. and abroad have used our system in the last five years for instruction, self-assessment and, in more limited numbers, for end-of-clerkship evaluations. The continued collection of data from thousands of student case interactions has allowed refinement in the scoring of the simulations. Scoring approaches have concentrated on replicating expert global judgments of examinee case management strategies. One method uses judgment modeling techniques to assess optimum waste for individual actions, and another explicitly captures and applies expert policies regarding case management.

Enhanced case authoring tools have been developed that capitalize on the database of existing cases using graphical and highly indexed computer-aided design tools to streamline case authoring. The simulation system has been rewritten using state-of-the-art techniques, including a graphical interface, the potential for integration of digital audio and video, and object-oriented database and programming.

Current activities are driven by the strategic plan for enhancement of United States Medical Licensing Examination (USMLE) adopted by the National Board and The Federation of State Medical Boards (FSMB) in 1995. The Phase I Implementation Plan, approved by the USMLE parent boards in March and April 1996, calls for the implementation of case simulations in the Step 3 Examination as early as 1998. At the same time, all three step examination multiple-choice question components will be converted to computer administration using an adaptive sequential testing model. This will allow Steps 1 and 2 to be shortened to one day each from the current two-day length. This rapid move to computerization of USMLE has been made possible by the emergence of secure, large scale computer-based testing networks. The National Board has entered into an agreement with a computer-based testing vendor to enhance its delivery system to meet the needs of our testing program.

As a prototype of our future program, the National Board and the Federation of State Medical Boards converted the Special Purpose Examination (SPEX) to computer in September 1995. This program is provided to the state medical boards to assess general medical knowledge. It is used by the states when they require an examination for licensure by endorsement of another state's license or by states that are looking for documentation of adequate knowledge as part of disciplinary proceedings. We are also well on the way to implementing computer-based testing programs for several of our client organizations, with current implementation dates for these programs between June 1996 and early 1998.

With this background overview of our voyage of nearly 30 years, let me highlight a few of the lessons we've learned from this experience (Figure 2).

Figure 2

Lessons from the NBME Voyage

- Measures are more difficult to create than methods.
- When all else fails, trust expert instincts.
- Test delivery is more technologically demanding than test development.
- The temptation to do it yourself can be overwhelming.
- Patience is a virtue and vision is essential.

First, measures are more difficult than methods. While the technology of computer-based testing is always the first topic of conversation, our experience at the National Board has proved over and over that the technologic problems are far less daunting than the measurement problems. Our simulation model was conceptually complete by the late 1970s. We have made many refinements, updating the model to take advantage of emerging technologies: virtual disks and Random Access Memory (RAM) in 1984, analogue video disks in 1985, digital audio and video in 1994, object-oriented programming in 1993—all these are examples of technological changes. However, the basic logical structure of the system has been stable for many years.

Appearances have changed (Figure 3) but the basic structure of the simulation engine has not.

Figure 3

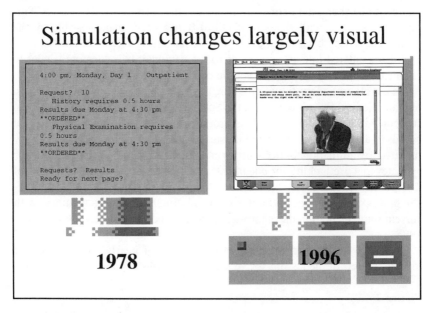

Simulation changes largely visual

1978

1996

The dumb terminal of 1978, completely character based and requiring input of coded numbers from the printed index, has given way to a networked personal computer running under Microsoft Windows® and exploiting its graphical interface. It includes full motion segments as part of the patient introduction, free-text entry on a mock order sheet, and iconic representation of time and location. But, as you may recall from the earlier time line, scoring research has continued throughout the developmental time line. The research has not just been on the incremental exploitation of technology; rather, it has required repeated creative approaches to solve specific recalcitrant problems. In particular, scoring and simulation design must proceed hand in hand, each informing the other.

The three major approaches to scoring have built less upon one another than upon the weaknesses discovered with the predecessor scoring method. Initial scoring methods adapted PMP scoring systems. As with PMPs, this system rewarded thoroughness rather than efficiency and often scored good novices higher than highly competent experts. The Rasch partial-credit model allowed better use of information gathered about timing and sequencing of actions and depended on item difficulty to weight the various actions. Separate categories for very risky actions were segregated from actions that were allowed to compensate for one another. The latter approach represented a conceptual shift toward combining quantitative and qualitative data in scoring the case simulations. This was the first step toward our current rule based, case logical approach. Probably the most significant step forward in scoring strategy was the move to capturing and replicating expert judgment about total case management. This approach has increased the precision with which the computer-generated scores can replicate the judgments of experts about the performances.

The NBME has consistently found the challenges in the development of innovative testing methods to lie primarily in the scoring arena. Complex test stimuli result in complex responses which require complex models to capture and appropriately combine information from the test to create a valid score. It is amazing to me how many complex "testing" simulation systems have been developed in the last decade, each *without* a scoring system. We strongly advocate the reliance on expert judgment about performances rather than items in creating scoring approaches. Finally, case specificity and the resultant limited generalized ability of small sets of cases cannot be ignored. Long tests are generally required when more complex test stimuli are used.

Answering the question "what are we measuring" with a new test is extremely difficult. I am not sure that we are even very certain of exactly what it is that we measure with our current tests. Despite two large field trials demonstrating that case simulations measured something distinct from MCQ and PMP tests, experts on our CBT advisory panel were troubled that we could not present data that convincingly defined the distinct attributes. This posture was taken primarily by test-development-wise physicians on the panel who perhaps overestimated the potential for precision in this field of research. The eminent psychometrician on that panel argued that whatever was being measured that was distinct was clinically important. He based his argument on the extensive involvement of physician experts at every stage of test development, content definition, case design, case authoring, case approval, scoring key development, key validation, research design, and evaluation of research results. He further argued that if the tasks presented by the cases and the scoring criteria were judged clinically relevant by these experts, and the research data showed them to be measuring a distinct attribute, then that attribute must be relevant to clinical practice. In effect, he argued that common sense is essential in the interpretation of validity evidence for the new method. He also argued we should not attempt to substitute quantitative research findings for the instincts of our panels of experts.

Throughout the history of our CBT project, applying technology to the task of test method development has not been easy. In fact, we have had to work hard to keep up with rapidly developing and evolving technology in selecting tools to solve our unique problems. It has always seemed that just as we squeezed a technology to solve a problem, a new technology emerged that solved the problem without contortions. It is easy to forget, however, the requirements for successful delivery of a technology-based test. Whether testing a few hundred or tens of thousands of examinees, the logistical challenge of providing a suitable testing environment with standardized test conditions is immense. It is easy to buy a few of the latest PCs or peripheral devices for your development environment and tempting to do so to allow the latest and best tools to be applied in solving your problems, but cost becomes significant when it is scaled up to the delivery system. Providing state-of-the-art and updating it frequently is likely to make a delivery system economically non-viable. I have seen more extremely creative simulation systems die in the last 15 years because no one would invest in the technology required to run them than for any other reason.

Our experience indicates that computer-based testing should target well defined, standard technology that is available economically. Only in this manner is it likely that large-scale test administration systems will be available at a defensible cost. Keep an eye on the cutting edge for future development but don't doom your CBT plans by requiring a delivery system that will not be available.

Most of you assembled here possess expertise in evaluation for certification. To make a technology-based testing program work, you need equivalent expertise in technology — both at the hardware and software systems development levels. In addition, you must be able to effectively design, construct, finance, market, and manage a technology-based delivery system. Few of you are experts in technology or in the creation and management of a technology-based delivery network; neither are your organizations. The NBME learned this truth the hard way. I have already described our aborted effort to create our own delivery system. Once again, the temptations presented by full control and specification of delivery system characteristics are alluring, but there is more to running a technology-based delivery system than defining what it would ideally look like. Our lack of skill in developing a sound and realistic business plan cost us millions of dollars and delayed our use of computer-based testing by years. Similarly the control offered by internally developing your computer-based testing system is attractive, but I have never seen an internally developed software system delivered on time or within budget. If Microsoft® has trouble doing it, what makes you think you can?

In retrospect, the NBME should have leaned more heavily on external expert help in these areas. While we have developed considerable expertise in these areas over the years, it has come at the cost of tremendous prolongations of the development cycle for CBT and has increased the cost.

I am convinced that the emergence of effective, secure networks for test delivery is the greatest single factor making computer-based testing at long last realistic. Our institutional plan is to shun the development of our own test delivery network, depending instead on strategic partners to focus their expertise on that task. Similarly, we have learned over the years that it is more efficient to use available technology resources by licensing proven software for part or all of our systems than to build everything from scratch.

The payback for our mistakes is the accumulation of considerable expertise in these areas after many years of effort. I doubt if the gain was worth the cost, however, and encourage you to seek assistance from those who are experienced in planning for computer-based testing.

Finally, patience is a virtue and vision is essential. Computer-based testing is different—it requires many changes in dearly held assumptions. The time-honored roomful of examinees and on-looking proctors, No. 2 pencils, the group experience of preparing for and taking a test—all these become obsolete with computer-based testing. In addition to the usual resistance to change, many stakeholders in high stakes examination programs will have particular reasons for concern. Older board members who are less likely to be computer literate will consider the medium to be an unfair disadvantage despite evidence that it is not. Psychometricians will be unhappy with changes in assumptions about acceptable reliability and new methods of analyzing scores. Test developers know how to oversee the writing of multiple-choice questions, creating effective simulations requires a totally different set of skills. Each of these groups, and others as well, will find reason after reason to defer, delay or otherwise obstruct movement toward computer-based testing. Each group will cite the failures of technology to keep up with imagination. I have heard them say it before: "We have been talking about computer-based education and computer-based testing for years and nothing has ever come of it." The net effect of the natural conservatism in our profession and the particular changes required by CBT will result in progress that is always slower than advocates imagine in their worst dreams.

Our advice to those advocating the use of technology-based evaluation is to maintain the vision of what you hope to accomplish. Throughout the years of disappointing delays in use of case simulations, the NBME has continued to be motivated by its belief that MCQ exams are just not enough, that the essential characteristics of clinical safety and efficacy cannot be reduced to five options. And perseverance is also essential. Time lines drag on and implementation plans always seem to take years rather than months.

In his voyages, Ulysses, as reported by Homer in the *Odyssey*, met many challenges. You may remember his encounter with the Sirens, luring with their songs to certain death. He survived by plugging the ears of his crew and instructing them to bind him to the mast of the ship as they sailed by the Sirens. Since its earliest days computer technology has sung the Siren song of potential. Our lives will all be better, teaching will be revolutionized, we will be able to test more effectively. For decades these promises have been unfulfilled and have, in fact, lured many to disaster. Few robots clean our houses even today. Computer-based instruction languished for decades without catching on and the National Board's CBT project took a ten-year detour from its initial implementation plan. However, I believe we are now past the Sirens' shores and we have survived Scylla and Charybdis and, like Ulysses, our journey is near its end. Our ship is on the shores of Ithaca. Computer-based testing is a reality. Hundreds of thousands of individuals take high stakes, computer administered tests each year. Hundreds are being tested as we sit here today. The final success of technology-based evaluation is now ready to deliver on its promises to promote a new era of evolutionary improvement in assessment.

During my 13 years of association with the NBME computer-based testing project, I have often sympathized with Christopher Columbus whose diary of the first voyage notes the dissatisfaction of many with the tedium of the long voyage.

"Here the people could stand it no longer and complained of the long voyage; but the Admiral cheered them as best he could, holding out good hope of the advantages they would have."

(*Journal of the First Voyage,* October 10, 1492)

And, like Columbus, we at the National Board have held out the good hope of advantages to be had through computer-based testing. Today, however, Shakespeare's advice in *Julius Caesar*, Act 14.3, is more apt.

"There is a tide in the affairs of men, which, when taken at the flood, leads on to fortune; omitted, all the voyage of their life is bound in shallows and in miseries. We must take the current when it serves, or lose our ventures."

Testing in our profession must now recognize the tide of technology-based assessment and take the current where it serves. Otherwise, all the voyage of our institutional lives will be bound in shallows and misery. I wish you bon voyage.

Virtual Reality Environments in Medicine

Col. Richard M. Satava, M.D., FACS
and
Lt. Cmdr. Shaun B. Jones, M.D.
Advanced Research Projects Agency - DSO

Ever since the inception of the serious application of virtual environments (VE) by pioneers at NASA-Ames,[1] the University of North Carolina, Chapel Hill, and the Human Interface Technology Lab (University of Washington, Seattle),[2] there have been examples of medical education and training through simulation. The three major applications are 1) individual anatomic education and training, 2) medical crisis planning and training, and 3) medical virtual prototyping. In the first of these, the obvious parallel between the surgeon and the pilot, each requiring repeated and prolonged opportunities to practice life-threatening situations, led to early efforts for development of surgical simulators. Currently, pilots successfully acquire a great majority of their training in flight simulators.

For the second application, it became apparent that there existed a parallel between military battlefield training (such as used with SIMNET, NPSNET, and DIS), and the need to train for combat casualty care or for civilian disaster management. The power of using "mission rehearsal" for military combat in a VE was proven by the training that resulted in the overwhelming success of the Gulf War.

The third application has recently resulted in the initiation of a number of projects using VE as a virtual prototyping tool to design medical instruments, equipment, and entire operating rooms, not only for the refinement of form, fit and function, but also as a potential environment to test, evaluate and train upon equipment before it has been built. The latter is a direct analogy to the Boeing 777 program, in which pilots practiced upon a simulator of the 777 while the aircraft was being built; when the first aircraft left the assembly line, the pilots had over 1000 hours of simulated "flight time." Although many other examples could be cited, most would fit within these three fundamental categories.

121

Substituting Virtual for Real Environments

The use of VE as a metaphor or enhancement for real life situations reflects the integration of a 3-D anatomic image into a telepresence surgery console (Figure 1) as a virtual environment.

Figure 1

Telepresence surgery surgeon's console.
Courtesy of Philip Green, SRI International.

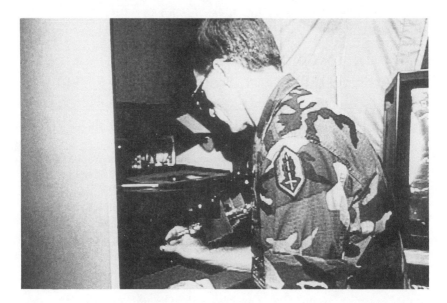

This provides the opportunity to do pre-operative planning of many possible procedures along with long-term prediction of the many possible outcomes.[3] (This is distinct from "augmented reality," in which the real and virtual environments are simultaneously displayed, often through a see-through head mounted display.) With telepresence surgery, in which surgery is performed on a virtual image of the real world in the display of the central console workstation,[4] the real image can be replaced with an identical computer-generated image, providing the opportunity to test, train, or evaluate the replica of the real world object(s) on the same input device as would be used for performing the real task. In a similar fashion, instead of using a graphic model of anatomy, patient specific data from imaging such as computed-axial tomography (CT scan), magnetic resonance imaging (MRI) or ultrasound can be used to render a patient specific virtual model (Figure 2) for planning and practicing a surgical procedure on the telepresence surgery console.

Figure 2

Patient specific knee from the "Visible Human" project dataset.
Courtesy of Dr. Scott Delp, MusculoGraphics, Inc.

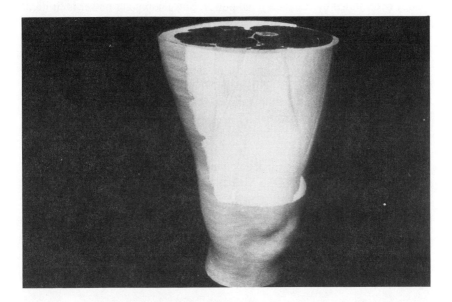

Once the results of the practiced surgical procedure are complete, the newly changed anatomy can be analyzed for the effects of the surgery over time, in essence predicting the results of the proposed surgery before the operation is performed.[5] As an example, a representation of a specific patient's knee from a CT scan can have a tendon reimplantation "performed;" once completed the patient's knee can be "walked" to see the results of the operation on the gait. Using the proper algorithms, the knee can be walked for years to predict the long-term results of that specific surgery.

The Question of "Realism"

The appearance of "realism," which can convey the impression of "presence" in a virtual environment, is related to fidelity and quantity of sensory input. Early research into cognition and perception for simulators provided anecdotal evidence that the realism of a simulation is related directly to the amount or number of the five senses incorporated into the simulation, and that the relationship was logarithmic, not linear. For example, if a second sensory input such as sound was added to a visual representation, it was four times more realistic, not just twice as realistic.

The most widely accepted explanation for this phenomenon is based on the neurophysiologic principles of recruitment and synergism, the biologic equivalent of the whole is greater than the sum of the parts. At the current state-of-the-art in creating VE, the fidelity of a given sensory input (such as vision) is mainly determined by computational power. Since computer power is finite, it must be shared among the multiple sensory inputs within a given VE.[6] There are, thus, very practical considerations when designing a VE regarding the sensory input. Will the VE be more "realistic" if the computational power is used to increase the visual fidelity (Figure 3), or should there be slightly less visual fidelity but an additional second input, such as sound or touch, to enhance the feeling of "presence." Until computational power is nearly unlimited, this basic trade-off will be required in every VE.

Figure 3

High visual fidelity of anatomy of a patient's chest.
Courtesy of Robert Butler, Glaxo Virtual Anatomy.

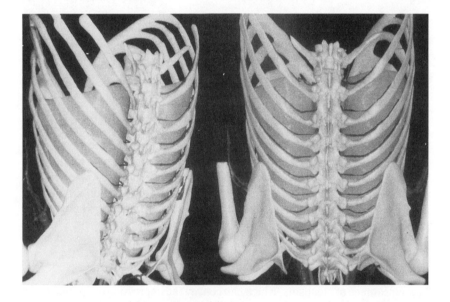

Inputs Other Than Visual and Auditory

Visual and auditory inputs are relatively sophisticated. However, the use of the sense of touch remains at a relatively primitive level, and the senses of olfaction and taste have not been implemented at all. "Touch" is a much greater challenge than either visual or auditory inputs. "Touch" is actually a combination of more than 20 anatomically discrete neurosensors that convey component information such as pressure, vibration, shear and microshear, two point discrimination, temperature, et cetera. It is no wonder that only modest gains have been achieved in "touch" using force reflection or simple tactile arrays or vibratory displays.[7,8]

It is unknown how important olfaction is to realism[9], but there are two interesting observations that suggest importance. First is the fact that even the most evanescent smell of a specific odor can trigger an enormous rush of memories and emotion. Second, in terms of brain sensory mapping, the second largest amount of brain volume is dedicated to olfaction, with the entire inferior surface of the frontal lobe producing numerous connections directly into those parts of the brain which appear important for emotion. The olfactory component seems to be a powerful subliminal sense, and its true contribution to realism in the sense of our discussion today, is yet to be understood.[10]

On the other hand, taste seems of limited importance, both physically and in terms of the quantity of brain tissue devoted to primary sensation. It can be expected to have a rather limited place unless further research reveals a greater role in daily interaction with our environment in developing of VE.

It is interesting to speculate on the use of synesthesia (replacing one sensory input with another) to convey a particular facet of a VE.[11] This is done commonly in some simple VEs, in which collision detection between two objects is signaled not by touch but by sound.

Integration of Virtual Environments for Medical Training

The basic challenge here is to integrate the three types of medical virtual environments, using many sensory inputs to increase "realism" yet optimize real time interactivity. The military has a need for training medics and physicians in battlefield combat casualty care, and three types of VE are needed to fully train for the battlefield. Current methodology for training in life saving is through a number of real world simulations called training exercises. To practice the basic skills of patient stabilization and wound care, animal models are used (e.g., production of gunshot wounds to the legs of goats). For triage, expensive field training exercises are conducted on "moulaged" soldiers. (Incidentally, there is no opportunity to practice the wound care or surgery on the "wounded" moulaged patients.) Finally, the evacuation of wounded casualties is conducted through medivac training exercises. While admitting that there is no VE that is even close to resembling the real world, it must be admitted that the current method of training as described above is disjointed. The training exercise, for example, does not allow for actual practice of the basic skills (e.g., inserting chest tubes or debridement of wounds in moulaged soldiers). The exercise also lacks the realism of true combat casualty care. One scenario which the military is investigating attempts to integrate all the above components into a series of seamless transitions in a VE.

A Military Scenario for Training in Combat Casualty Care

A description of the early exploratory phases of one integrated program for combat casualty care can be provided as follows: The individual medic is a member of a squad (or platoon) of soldiers inserted into a networked, synthetic battlefield (Figure 4).

Figure 4

Virtual medic and wounded soldier in virtual battlefield.
Courtesy Dr. Norman Badler, University of Pennsylvania.

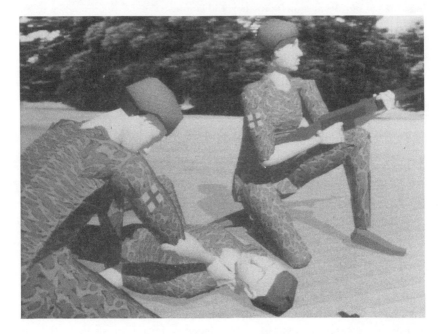

The insertion is accomplished by using a device referred to as the I-Port or Individual Portal into the VE[12] (Figure 5).

Figure 5

The I-Port for virtual environments.
Courtesy of Dr. Stephen Jacobsen, Sarcos, Inc.

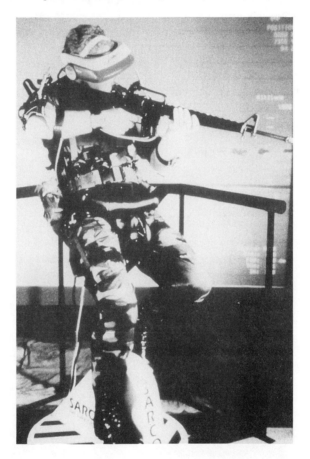

The medic wears a head-mounted display and an exoskeleton (to track his motions) and either sits on an exercycle device or runs on a treadmill. The soldier's figure (avatar) would then appear in the virtual battlefield. When the medic waves his hand, the avatar waves; when the medic pedals the exercycle or runs on the treadmill, the avatar moves through the environment. When a soldier is "wounded" in the VE, the soldier's avatar falls down and a symbolic "wound" appears in the correct anatomic area. If multiple soldiers are wounded, the medic must practice triage, that is, pedal or treadmill over to the soldier with the most serious wounds first. When the medic arrives at the side of the wounded soldier, the scene must change from a generic wounded soldier to the specific wound that was sustained. This can be accomplished by the medic "looking down" at the soldier. "Looking down" will switch the VE from a networked terrain-based environment to the local anatomic database, with an appropriate wound created upon the anatomic part. When looking down, the medic will see a leg with a gunshot wound to the femur, with associated surgical instruments and bandages to do wound debridement and packing[13] (Figure 6).

Figure 6

Virtual gunshot wound to the thigh, current state of the art.
Courtesy of Dr. Scott Delp, MusculoGraphics, Inc.

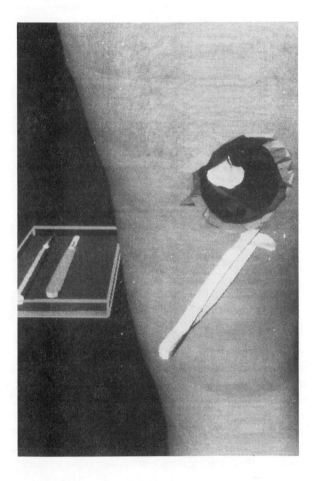

When the medic completes first aid and stabilization, the casualty must be evacuated from the battlefield. The medic then "looks up" and the database is switched back to the terrain VE. Within the terrain environment will be other medical equipment; some is part of the standard inventory (e.g., medivac helicopters), while other equipment comprises virtual prototypes, such as the Life Support for Trauma and Transport (LSTAT or Trauma Pod), the new Armored Ambulance or perhaps even a concept model of the Medical Forward Armored Surgical Telepresence (MEDFAST) vehicle.[14] Working together with other medics or soldiers, the casualty will be placed on a litter or LSTAT and loaded into the medivac helicopter for evacuation. To enhance realism of the scenario, not only will there be visual and auditory input, but also preliminary, relatively primitive attempts at tactile input (to feel the wound or surgical instruments), and olfactory input (to smell smoke, gunpowder, or medical odors). This integrated scenario offers something that is impossible today — it provides in a single continuous simulation the entire sequence of events that are required to locate, triage, treat and evacuate a casualty. There will be no need for the expensive logistics of a field exercise, the wounding of animals, or the mobilization of ambulances and helicopters. And, of course, the training can be repeated until perfected.

Challenges for Medical Virtual Environments

Even such a brief scenario as described above (soldier is wounded, medic does triage and gives first aid, casualty is evacuated to helicopter) is extraordinarily complex and involves multiple levels of integration.

At the highest level is the difficulty of integrating the networked terrain VE with the local anatomic VE. Questions include, for example, how will the medic be represented in the networked environment while working in the local mode, how will changes from one VE database be translated to another, or what is the impact on network traffic. For representing the avatar in the VE, there are issues of how articulated does the figure need to be, what is the minimum of sensors required to accurately translate motion and actions, how to perform collaborative tasks such as lifting a litter, should there be semi-autonomous or autonomous behaviors, or what level of detail of the hand is required to perform manipulative tasks. For the input devices such as the I-Port, exoskeleton or the position sensors, the question of accuracy and sensitivity of the sensors, level of encumbrance of the input device, ability to perform full range of actions and tasks, are but a few of the technical challenges to providing a convincing and realistic simulation.

As these technical problems are being faced, there is an even greater task: to reinvent what the content of the training should be. It is essential to understand precisely what the new technology brings to the educational experience and the difference between the interactive, immersive environment and previous media formats (e.g., slides, books, blackboards). In order to exploit the educational power of the VE to the fullest, the uniqueness of the medium must be used to provide a new dimension to the educational content. Using the same old educational material in VE is foolish since the learning experience will be essentially unchanged. Lesson plans should capitalize upon full immersive 3-D effects with real time interactivity (the difference from previous media—the technology difference or ΔT) to provide an educational perspective not otherwise possible (the difference in the educational experience or ΔE).

An example from the above scenario might be the fully interactive "virtual anatomy" of the wounded leg. ΔT is the infinite perspective and change of a fully 3-D image that permits the student to explore around, between and inside the tissues. The ΔE is the freedom through self-discovery to obtain a perception and understanding of the anatomic relationships and ballistic effects not otherwise possible by reading or viewing a CD-ROM. Perhaps the added technical value (ΔT) is the continuity of the entire combat casualty experience. A curriculum should be designed that includes the tempo and continuity (the ΔE) of casualty care. Understanding the technology advantage and applying the technology to the educational content is one of the most exciting challenges of creating and learning in a VE.

Conclusions

For over a decade virtual environments have been used for education and training in scenarios other than flight simulation. Some virtual environments provide extensive worlds using terrain databases to explore and interact, while others are complex objects, (the "Visible Human" Project, for example), scaled to human proportion and requiring very little navigation. All types of VE have in common a high level of interactivity and immersion, permitting an infinite number of possible views, interactions, and reactions. A major technical challenge is integration of the various contexts of virtual environments to provide a more real world experience from individual task to cooperative training. Of equal importance is understanding the technical advantage of a given virtual environment, and designing educational content to capitalize on this uniqueness. The goal is to provide learning experiences significantly greater than is possible in current educational and training experiences.

Bibliography

1. Ellis SR. *Pictoral Communication in Virtual and Real Environments (2nd Ed.)*, Washington, DC: Taylor and Francis, 1993.

2. Barfield W, Furness TA. *Virtual Environments and Advanced Interface Design*. New York: Oxford University Press, 1995.

3. Piper S, Delp S, Rosen J, Fisher S. A Virtual Environment System for Simulation of Leg Surgery. *Proc of Stereoscopic Display and Applications II*, SPIE 1991;1457:188-196.

4. Green PS, Hill JW, Jensen JF, Shah A. Telepresence Surgery. *IEEE Engineer in Med in Biol* 1995: 14:324-329.

5. Delp SL, Zajac FR. Force and moment gathering capacity of lower limb muscles before and after tendon lengthening. *Clin Ortho Related Research;* 1992;284:247-259.

6. Sheridan TB. Musings on telepresence and virtual presence. *Presence* 1992;1:120-125.

7. Salisburg JK, Brock D, Massie T, Swarup N, Zilles C. Haptic rendering: Programming touch interaction with virtual objects. *Proc of ACM 1995 Symposium on Interactive 3-D Graphics*, Monterey, CA, April 1995.

8. Burdea G and Coifett P. Touch and Force Feedback, in *Virtual Reality Technology*. New York: John Wiley & Sons, Inc. (Chapter 3:81-116) 1994.

9. Satava RM. The Third Hand and Missing Nose, in *Proc of Medicine Meets Virtual Reality - III*, San Diego, CA, January 1994.

10. Kruger MW. Olfactory Stimuli in Virtual Reality Applications. In Satava RM, Morgan K et al, Ed. *Interactive Technology and the New Medical Paradigm for Health Care*. Washington, DC: ISO Press; 1995 pp 180-81.

11. Addison R. DETOUR: Brain Deconstruction Ahead. In Satava RM, Morgan K et al Ed. *Interactive Technology and the New Medical Paradigm for Health Care*. Washington, DC: IOS Press; 1995 pp 1-4.

12. Jacobsen SC. Personal communication.

13. Delp S. Personal communication.

14. Kaplan K, Hunter I, Durlach NI, Schodek DL, Rattner D. A Virtual Environment for a Surgical Room of the Future. In Satava RM, Morgan K et al, Ed. *Interactive Technology and the New Medical Paradigm for Health Care*. Washington, DC: IOS Press, 1995 pp 161-167.

Discussion

Col. Richard M. Satava, M.D. (Advanced Research Projects Agency): Great toys, but the key to Virtual Reality simulations and why you are the absolute key to the future is that it is the medical content that makes the difference. No matter how good the toys are, if you don't design a good educational program and an evaluation system, all the technology is absolutely worthless. I give you all a challenge. What I hope you learned today is that the technology is ready. Dr. Melnick has shown the experience is here to leverage off the technology. I would like you all today, each of the members of the boards, to put a stake in the ground. Place the stake at ten years from today and the flag on the top says, "We test physicians using simulations." That gives us five years for our technology to increase. A Howard Moore cycle is 18 months, a doubling of the order of magnitude for improvement in technology every 18 months; that is the basis of the information age, and the basis of our computer-based technology. It can be expected to continue. So, within the next five years, the technology will be ready to begin testing technical and haptic skills for a procedure-related physician. That leaves five years for physicians to practice on the new simulators. Ten years from today we would be able to begin to actually test physicians on the simulators. If you do not do this, we may languish for the next twenty to thirty years. If there is a leadership role played by the boards, then we will be perceived by the industry that it is worthwhile to invest the money in this effort just as they did in the aviation industry. The aviation industry built simulators because they knew the pilots would be tested. We do not have such a requirement in medicine. I know this is a bold step, but I can tell you from the younger physicians that talk to me, that you, meaning those who are responsible for education and certification, are being viewed in one of two camps whether you like it or not.

Either you are a visionary or you are an obstructionist. You need to grasp the technologies that are native and intuitive to young physicians today, those which I showed you. These are not my perceptions but those of younger researchers, and the physicians that are coming to the training programs today, bringing questions to me and saying, "This is my world, where is it?" We need your experience. We need your stringent evaluation and guidance in order to go forward correctly into the future.

David Troxel, M.D., (American Board of Pathology): Several of the presenters today have alluded to The Visible Human Project. I suddenly realized I know little bits and pieces about it, but I do not have a good overview of it. I suspect other members of the audience may not either. I wonder if Dr. Satava or someone else would like to address in a few minutes an overview about, not only the project, but its availability.

Dr. Satava: In 1994, the National Library of Medicine (NLM) was able to acquire a cadaver which was sliced into 1,874 slices. Using CT (computerized tomography) and MRI (Molecular Resonance Imaging), there are now three full data sets at one millimeter apart, i.e., with one millimeter resolution. The three sets are CT, MRI, and cross-sectional slides, all on digitalized data. The data can be reassembled in any direction you would care to, in essence our very first virtual human being. It is up to us to take the data that is available about this person and reconstruct it in any way we wish. The great power is that The Visible Human dataset can serve as a standard. Every time a helical CT scan is done on a patient, the data can be used in the same way that we did with The Visible Human. Patient-specific data can be manipulated to do education, training, pre-operative planning, intraoperative stereotactic assistance, and even prognostication.

The point is that we now have digitalized information equivalent to a real human being. In the not too distant future every patient can be represented as an information equivalent. I think this is the power of the information age.

Donald E. Melnick, M.D. (National Board of Medicine Examiners): I might just add that the data from The Visible Human Project are available. I do not have the Worldwide Website address but if you use your search engine and look for Visible Human, there is an NLM Web page that describes the licensing requirements, and the media in which The Visible Human data are available. It is something that is being made available for a variety of uses.

Dr. Satava: It's not only made available, it is free, because it was a government funded project. But I would caution you that it is 45 megabytes of information. If you want to download it, it will take approximately two-and-a-half days of continuous connection.

For those of you who are in research, there are ten sections from the top to the bottom on diskettes, available at $100 per disk, and this is instantaneously downloaded for you. If there is ever any question, just ask Dr. Michael Ackerman at the National Library of Medicine, the conference keynote speaker.

Dr. Satava: If I could just make one more comment. One of the keys, as I said, is the content. If you look at the technology, when we started with pencil and paper in books, we had a two-dimensional technology. We added a third dimension when we added multimedia and video. Virtual reality adds a fourth dimension, time. Thus three dimensions of space plus time. The key here is the change in technology, adding the extra dimension of technology. We need to design our examinations by using the advantage, the ΔE if you will, the educational advantage, based on the difference between the old and the new technology. The educational change, the increased value of the educational experience, should reflect the difference between the old technology and the new technology—the three-dimensional space. The availability to explore from infinite perspectives is what a virtual world provides. Your educational tools should take advantage of this new perspective, not be just another pen and paper-based technology.

TODAY'S OPPORTUNITIES AND TOMORROW'S POSSIBILITIES

PART

6

Today's Opportunities and
Tomorrow's Possibilities

Discussion

Concluding Remarks

Today's Opportunities and Tomorrow's Possibilities

Roger C. Kershaw
Educational Testing Service

The Educational Testing Service (ETS) has been in the forefront of computer-based testing (CBT) for many years. Indeed, adaptive testing, one of the key concepts enabling, if not propelling, CBT as a viable alternative to paper-based test administrations was prototyped by ETS research staff in 1978. It was then that Dr. Fred Lord developed and published his first papers on Item Response Theory which formed the basis for adaptive testing. All of the college admissions testing programs at ETS and most of the certification tests base their assessment models on Dr. Lord's work. ETS currently has nine testing programs delivered or about to be delivered by computers in testing centers around the world. These programs are targeted today toward graduate school admissions testing (GRE General Test already in place, the Graduate Management Admission Test coming on-line late in 1997 and the Test of English as a Foreign Language to be released in 1998). Many credentialing tests are also on-line today, developed by ETS and its subsidiary, The Chauncey Group International. The most prominent exemplar of these examinations is the licensing of registered and practical nurses (National Council Licensure Examination) for all 62 state boards of nursing in the U.S. under the auspices of the National Council of State Boards of Nursing.

The Advent of Adaptive Testing Technology

Although research began in the mid-1970s, the first national computer-based testing programs at ETS began live in 1992 with the Graduate Record Examination linear test, a computerized version of the paper test designed to collect information on the comparability of the paper exam and the CBT version.

139

At the same time, ETS introduced the Praxis Series of computerized tests for beginning teachers. After comparability had been established, these exams used adaptive testing techniques in the delivery and scoring. These adaptive tests and those that followed offered statisticians improved measurement precision over the ability range of the potential examinee population. Basically the adaptive test delivers items, calibrated by difficulty, to each examinee according to his or her ability level. Beginning with an item of average difficulty, the adaptive algorithm selects more difficult items if the examinee answers correctly and easier items when answers are incorrect. In some testing programs, item delivery is programmed to terminate after reaching the optimum precision on the ability estimate. This is commonly known as the stopping rule. The selection algorithm balances item delivery for content domain, item response styles, item overlap, and item exposure rates.

Adaptive testing experiences in examination programs for admissions purposes, where content knowledge has been traditionally measured in paper-based tests with scaled scores such as the 200 to 800 range, led the way for mastery testing techniques. In mastery testing, small groups of items are administered in a sequence of increasing difficulty until the stopping rules indicate that presenting the examinee with more "testlets" would not increase the value of assessment which is typically indicated as "pass" or "fail." In both the adaptive and mastery models fewer items are required to yield the same precision estimate of ability than are required in a linear test. In a linear test the examinees are required to answer questions that are obviously too easy for people of high ability or too hard for people of low ability.

Enabling Technologies

At the same time that measurement science provided justification from the statistical view, advances in technology provided the platform for computerized test delivery. For example, the personal computer, especially the graphical user interface, facilitated the economical delivery and ease of use required to serve adequately diverse populations of examinees sitting for examinations on a national scale. Local area networks provided the security and control mechanisms for test administrators to proctor multiple examinations in a testing center. Advances and economies in data communications permitted test sponsors and testing agencies to distribute test item pools internationally in a matter of days and return test results in a matter of minutes following completion of an examination. Sophisticated software and database systems for appointment reservations eliminated the need to register for tests weeks in advance of an examination. Of particular note were the hardware and software advances which allowed us to provide access to examinations for people with disabilities. Examples of these special accommodations were screen magnification for people with visual impairment, variable time limits for people with learning disabilities, and specialized keyboards for people with motor skill impairment.

Benefits of Computerized Examinations

The incentives to computerize the examinations were numerous and diverse. The most compelling, however, was the increased precision of the examination itself provided by adaptive testing. Convenience to examinees was highly attractive as well and had many dimensions including safe, comfortable and private facilities for test taking, shorter waiting period for appointments, faster reporting times, and continuous testing throughout the calendar year. Expanded service and marketing opportunities for the test sponsor through computer test delivery were important. Related products and services such as diagnosis and instruction on skill deficiencies could be offered to the examinee immediately following the examination. CBT offered significant advantages in improved security methods and facilities because paper forms of the examinations are not in circulation and the test is administered in a highly controlled environment.

Many researchers at ETS believe, however, that the opportunity to pursue new forms of assessment, beyond multiple-choice questions and essay tests, is the primary motivation for converting to CBT. In the section under tomorrow's possibilities, there is a discussion of the next generation of assessment methods.

Current and Best Practices

A quick look at the state-of-the-art today in CBT reveals several important and key elements in planning a nationwide, high stakes, computerized examination program. The components of a CBT are rather simple and obvious. In general, they are the same as administering a paper examination. There are crucial differences though in many areas. You need a process for **test creation**, a method for distribution of the exam (**test distribution**), a network of locations and a system to deliver the test (**the testing network**), and a method for reporting results to test takers and institutions interested in the results (**test results processing**).

Test Creation

Creating the test suitable for computer delivery is obviously the first step (after clearly setting the purpose of the test and high level test specification). It is not the purpose of this paper to describe the events in adaptive CBT test creation; however, a description of a typical set of events helps in appreciating the projections for estimated test completion time.

Assuming the test sponsor wishes to anchor the computerized test to prior paper tests in order to maintain comparability, there are two aspects: one establishes that the CBT version is comparable, to the degree necessary, to the paper test; and the other enables the score results of the CBT to be reported on the same metric scale as the paper test. Comparability test studies and item equating sets are the most common approaches to providing the statistical evidence required in these cases. If the measurement model selected is an adaptive or mastery model, item difficulty calibration using the Item Response Theory or the Rasch model is required. Recently, several new techniques have been proposed which obviate the need for specialized item calibration; however, certain test specifications must be met in order for these methods to be employed.

The next steps include statistical and test development activities required to expand the item pool and assemble the items into clusters of test items that meet test specifications. Typically, adaptive testing requires very large item pools in order for the item selection algorithm to deliver the optimum test to the examinee. Item pools on the order of 1500 to 2000 items per pool and two or more pools created per year are common. Because of these requirements and parallel activities that will be described later, converting a paper-based, linear examination to an adaptive CBT may take as little as six months and as much as twenty-four months.

Multiple-choice examinations currently are easier and faster to implement, primarily because the items that form the starting test pools exist in most cases. Essay item types are, as a rule, easy to implement as well, but scoring essay item types remains today as a labor intensive, relatively expensive activity and will continue to be until advancements in measurement and technology enable automated scoring.

If the test sponsor wishes to establish a new CBT examination, current practices include a formal job analysis to establish the skills and knowledge base required for mastery of the content domains in the profession. The test sponsor establishes the overall test specifications and the subject matter, and experts define the content domain. As in the case where a CBT examination is converted from a paper test, the steps from this point forward are similar but without the need to establish test and score comparability or concordance.

Item and test development activities for computerized tests differ significantly from paper-based tests. Paper-based test layout and composition can be performed by most commercial printing vendors. Preparation for computer delivery of tests, however, requires custom designed software integrated with the test delivery system at testing centers. Several commercial providers offer custom software systems that will facilitate the item and test creation process and even enable item pool assembly and test delivery. Experience has shown that these solutions are less than satisfactory for many test sponsors unless they have integrated the computer and manual systems required to administer high stakes, national examination programs. The same problem exists with commercial word processing, spreadsheet and statistical software sometimes used in the test creation process by small testing agencies. Most large testing agencies today have evolved to the use of highly integrated and automated systems for test creation, statistic analysis, examinee eligibility, appointment processing, test administration, test delivery, scoring and reporting.

Test Distribution

ETS and our delivery partner, Sylvan Prometric, have a method for electronic test pool delivery which ensures that the latest versions of the test are where they should be at the right time. Essentially, all test centers have all the latest tests on site. Updates to the network of testing centers occur approximately once per month when new exams are introduced, pretest items are rotated, or item pools are updated. Each testing program, however, has its own schedule for these periodic updates. Item pool data are created, encrypted and packaged at ETS, delivered electronically to Sylvan headquarters in Maryland, and distributed electronically to every center authorized to offer the test domestically and/or internationally. Some testing agencies have elected to download tests to test centers when an appointment for a particular test is made, and not keep the test resident at the test center. This approach has its advantages and could be a viable alternative to the approach that we have instituted.

The Testing Network

Creating test centers, unless contracted with an operational delivery vendor, are unquestionably the most cost and time intensive component of a CBT program. ETS and Sylvan Prometric established a worldwide capacity for over a million hours of testing this year, with centers dispersed geographically throughout the world based on clients' test taking populations. There are more than 260 test centers, operating up to twelve hours per day, and six days per week. Access for people with disabilities is a high priority in the layout and provisioning of these centers. To augment the site facilities, mobile testing centers currently operate along with established centers. The centers are connected electronically to Sylvan Prometric headquarters and to ETS. Within the next three years we anticipate test center capacity will more than double.

Test Results Processing

Paper-based testing systems focus on five basic functions: candidate registration, test center appointments by national test date, fee collection, answer sheet scanning, and score reporting. In computer-based testing, examinees can typically take the examination any day of the year, and appointment processing by telephone replaces the U.S. mail registration process. Fee collection for CBTs is preferably by credit card and taken at appointment time, although other forms of fee collection are offered. There are no answer sheets to process since the examinations are given by computer. Usually results are shown to the examinee on-screen immediately after the test, but some test sponsors reserve the right to report official test scores. In other words, all new systems and procedures must be developed for CBT purposes unless the test sponsor chooses to have the test delivery agency perform these tasks.

In addition to test development and statistical services, the CBT test delivery service provides generic capability for every testing function and offers a wide variety of options and choices for the test sponsor. A small sample of the options are listed in Figure 1.

Figure 1

Optional Test Delivery Services
Available at Test Centers

- Eligibility-based testing or walk-in testing.
- Security options such as finger printing and digital photo acquisition.
- Tutorials on computer use aimed at the novice computer user.
- Presentation of sample items.
- Mandatory and optional time breaks for examinees.
- Handwritten or computer-written essays.
- Retest policy options such as no retest within 90 days or blocking previously seen items.
- Linear, adaptive, mastery test models.
- Multiple-choice, essay and other constructed-response, or performance-based testing.
- Work simulations with reference tools and/or on-line access to databases.
- Human scoring of constructed-response items.
- Official results on screen or transmitted to test sponsor.
- Up to twenty item-response styles for multiple-choice tests.
- Pretest pool spiraling with existing item pools.
- Items with sophisticated graphics, animation, sound or video.
- Examinee biographical data collection.
- Examinee exit surveys.
- Electronic irregularity reports.

The administrative and delivery systems now in place offer these functions and many more services without the need for new development. Special features designed specifically for a particular examination program are also encouraged. Categorizing individual examinee results reporting is the most popular service. Every testing program will require specialized processing, security or statistical functions. Depending on the nature and extent of these requirements, the cost and time for development and implementation may increase.

Assuming the test sponsor has a clear understanding of the critical issues involved, one year is a feasible timeframe to create, distribute, and administer computerized examinations from initial test specification stages to national and international delivery. Many of the critical issues are the traditional test issues such as reliability, validity, fairness, test use, comparability across test forms and item pools, and the like. Test sponsors considering moving to CBT should have resolved these issues before embarking on computerization. Specifically for the computerized testing program, test sponsors will need to consider the psychometric model of choice for the credentialing examination (e.g., traditional test theory or item response theory); and the preparation required to implement the program.

Tomorrow's Possibilities

It is an exciting time for the assessment industry considering the possibilities ahead. Test sponsors should be aware that new forms of assessment that will leapfrog over current best practices in many areas are in research and development. Advances in multimedia technology presentation have enabled test developers to introduce more realistic assessments. In the credentialing arena, assessments are in place today that simulate workplace conditions and solicit performance-based, constructed-response solutions to problems. The current surge in development of new measures focuses on constructed-response item types and, more specifically, performance-based measures which go beyond multiple-choice questions. These performance measures typically include so-called authentic assessment and simulations that look more relevant to examinees and sponsors and complement conventional test questions in the kinds of skills they measure. For example in a listening comprehension test now in development, actual recordings of reading of item stems are played to the examinee through the use of the PC with sound capability. Recent developments in sophisticated scoring systems also lay the foundation for these new item styles. Natural language-parsing systems can score written essays, and have logical scoring systems that can analyze and score complex examinee-produced solutions to problems. There are exemplars of the new scoring system that illustrate the concept. The National Council of Architectural Registration Boards (NCARB) will begin in January 1997 to assess candidates for certification. The licensing examinations contain eight assessment components, including several objective-type mastery tests and several work simulations (referred to as "vignettes").

Other advances that enable these forecasts are faster and less expensive data communications methods such as digital networks (ISDN), CD-ROM technology, high capacity media storage devices, multimedia capable personal computers, object-oriented software, and software innovations such as Microsoft's® object-linking and embedding techniques.

While these technologies continue to emerge and mature, cost and development time remain prohibitive to many test sponsors; however, research and development in these directions show that it should be feasible to produce in a short time performance-based measures utilizing multimedia capabilities for national examinations.

Currently, research into advanced techniques for test creation also proceeds in exciting and most cost effective ways. These advances include item cloning methods, reusability of retired items, automated item pool assembly systems, repurposing of existing multimedia components and sophisticated graphical editing and display systems.

What test sponsors should be contemplating as they think about future examinations depends greatly on the purposes of the exam, the problems inherent in their current capabilities and the possibilities suggested by many of the conference presenters. I am always reminded that prescription without diagnosis is called malpractice, and would strongly recommend a focused analysis by a professional measurement organization before implementing a plan of action.

Discussion

Dorthea Juul, Ph.D. (American Board of Psychiatry & Neurology): I have a question about item banks. Using adaptive testing, how are new items calibrated and added into the item bank? If items are cloned, can it be assumed that the statistical properties that they had in a slightly different variation will be the same?

Roger C. Kershaw, (Educational Testing Service): I am not a psychometrician but maybe Dr. Isaac Bejar from the Educational Testing Service can help us; he is here. I will explain what we have done previously. Whenever converting from the kind of statistics captured traditionally in a paper-based test it is necessary to go through another pilot test study and perform a statistical analysis on the test items. It is not cheap and it is not easy, and certainly it is a long-term project.

Audience: When doing item cloning you go through the same kinds of statistical analytic steps as for other test items. In doing adaptive testing, I understand that it is fairly easy to get an estimate of total performance of a candidate. The only issue seems to be breadth of content to satisfy constituencies and to satisfy the courts. Except for the candidate who hugs the pass/fail line and wobbles around it, sooner or later I would guess that for that person most of the test questions presented are around that pass/fail line. When do you quit? How do you make the determination that this person is on the positive, i.e., passing side, or the negative, failing side? And a related question, if some of the test takers know what this game is all about, what is the psychic impact on the person who takes a longer test when everyone else has finished the test?

147

Mr. Kershaw: These are very good questions. The answer to the first question about when to stop testing is that the adaptive and mastery techniques are much better than a linear test for estimating a passing performance, but they are not perfect. In a continuous delivery of test items with a fairly large item pool and "testlets," the level of precision can be much more comfortable than is possible in any other test format; again, it is not perfect. In answer to the question about the public perception of a shorter test or a longer test, the best way to respond is a public information campaign to inform candidates about what these test techniques do; why the tests are fair; why one candidate may have a shorter test and another a longer test; and why we determined someone is essentially a high achiever or a lower achiever, or passes or fails. The problem will go away, I think, when the public becomes more aware and the constituencies that work with these test methods on an everyday basis are aware of their statistical characteristics.

Concluding Remarks

William H. Hartmann, M.D.
American Board of Pathology
and
Elliott L. Mancall, M.D.
Chair, Committee on Study of Evaluation Procedures

Dr. Hartmann: The conference has brought together people from a great variety of disciplines. The representatives of the boards, i.e., the Member Boards of the ABMS, have been well served by being here. I think the conference has been incredibly timely. There has been a lot of discussion, both within this room and in the exhibit hall, which has been mutually beneficial. I am here to suggest, to have the temerity to make the suggestion, that one of the outcomes of this conference should be the creation, by the Member Boards of ABMS, of a computer users group to deal effectively with the changes that are already upon us and are coming in computer-based testing. I would like the minutes of this conference to reflect the fact that there should be a users group formed by the boards to deal with the issue of computerization of examinations.

Dr. Mancall: Everyone with whom I have discussed Dr. Hartmann's suggestion has been enthusiastic. Hopefully the notion will get the blessing of the ABMS Executive Committee and move forward from there.

Finally, I want to thank all of you for coming to this conference. I personally found it an extraordinarily stimulating experience and I hope the rest of you did as well. We welcome you back to many future ABMS conferences.

Appendix I

Conference Participants

Faculty and Contributors

Michael J. Ackerman, PhD
Assistant Director for
    High Performance Computing &
    Communications
National Library of Medicine
Building 38
8600 Rockville Pike
Bethesda, MD 20894

Philip G. Bashook, EdD
Conference Coordinator
Director, Evaluation & Education
American Bd. Med. Specialties
1007 Church Street, Suite 404
Evanston, IL 60201-5913

Stephen M. Downs, MD, MS
Asst. Prof. Pediatrics &
    Biomedical Engineering
Div. of Community Pediatrics
CB7225 - Wing C
School of Medicine
University of North Carolina
Chapel Hill, NC 27599-7225

Charles P. Friedman, PhD
Asst. Dean for Medical Education
& Informatics Office of Educa-
    tional Development
School of Medicine
University of North Carolina
CB 7530 MacNider Building
Chapel Hill, NC 27599-7530

William H. Hartmann, MD
Executive Vice President
American Board of Pathology
One Urban Centre, Suite 690
4830 W. Kennedy Boulevard
P.O. Box 25915
Tampa, FL 33622-5915

Charles B. Johnston, PhD
Vice President Technology
Sylvan Prometric
2601 W. 88th St.
Bloomington, MN 55431

151

Lt. Comd. Shaun B. Jones, MD
Program Manager
Defense Research Projects
   Agency - DSO
3701 N. Fairfax Drive
Arlington, VA 22203

Roger C. Kershaw
Executive Director Software
   Engineering and Technology
   Information Systems
Educational Testing Services
Rosedale Road, Mail Drop #11D
Princeton, NJ 08541

Elliott L. Mancall, MD
Chairman, ABMS Committee on
   Study of Evaluation Procedures
Department of Neurology
Jefferson Medical School
1025 Walnut St., Suite 310
Philadelphia, PA 19107

Maurice J. Martin, MD
Mayo Clinic
Department of Psychiatry
200 First Street, S.W.
Rochester, MN 55905

Donald E. Melnick, MD
Senior Vice President
National Board of Medical
   Examiners
3750 Market Street
Philadelphia, PA 19104-3190

John J. Norcini, Ph.D.
Executive Vice President and
   Senior Assoc. to the President
American Board of Internal
   Medicine
University City Science Center
3624 Market Street
Philadelphia, PA 19104-2675

Gerald A. Rosen, EdD
Sylvan Technology Systems
3435 Central Avenue
Huntingdon Valley, PA 19006

Richard J. Rovinelli, PhD
Rovinelli Associates
501 Darby Creek Rd. - Ste. 16
Lexington, KY 40509

**Col. Richard M. Satava, MD,
   FACS**
Program Manager
Defense Research Projects
Agency-DSO
3701 N. Fairfax Drive
Arlington, VA 22203

Fred G. Smith, MD
Vice President
American Board of Pediatrics
111 Silver Cedar Court
Chapel Hill, NC 27514-1651

Anthony R. Zara, PhD
Director of Testing
National Council
   State Boards of Nursing
676 N. St. Clair, Suite 550
Chicago, IL 60611

Exhibitors

American Board of Family Practice

2228 Young Drive
Lexington, KY 40505

Over the past three years, the American Board of Family Practice has been developing a knowledge base in family medicine from which a computer-based system dynamically generates and presents patient simulations. As part of the demonstration there will be opportunity to discuss the following:

- The goals of the computer-based assessment project.
- The process used to achieve these goals.
- A description of the family practice knowledge base.
- The anticipated advantages of the computer-based assessment system.
- The anticipated generalizability of the computer-based assessment system.

American Board of Internal Medicine

University City Science Center
3624 Market Street
Philadelphia, PA 19104-2675

The ABIM designs and develops integrated item banking, item printing, and computerized examination software for its own use. The non-adaptive "Self-Evaluation Process" is its most recent computer-based examination.

American Board of Pathology

P.O. Box 25915
Tampa, FL 33622-5915

The exhibit will allow you to utilize the computer system employed by the American Board of Pathology for the subspecialty examinations in 1995. There will be a descriptive brochure of the system functions available. Each viewer should leave with an understanding of how this successful system can be used in your certification examination.

American Board of Pediatrics

111 Silver Cedar Court
Chapel Hill, NC 27514-1651

The American Board of Pediatrics will demonstrate its Program for Renewal of Certification in Pediatrics - Computer (PRCP-C). PRCP-C is administered by computer at home or at any other convenient location. There are three components: Knowledge, Diagnosis, and Management, all of which will be demonstrated and available for "hands on use."

American Board of Radiology

Suite 6800
5255 E. William Circle
Tucson, AZ 85711

This is a prototype workstation being evaluated for recertification, primary certification, or certification for advanced qualification (CAQ). The design supports: (1) customization based on specialty areas and experience level; (2) collection of data on usage, question difficulty, and subject performance; (3) randomizing question selection and modifying question format; and (4) multimedia content display. Use of all-digital media provides highest possible image resolution and flexible image manipulation, including both still and motion images, and management of screen "real estate" when multiple images or studies are pertinent to a question.

The Chauncey Group International
Rosedale Road
Princeton, NJ 08540

Innovative item types, precise measurement of candidates' abilities, and candidate convenience are just a few of the advantages that computer-based testing can provide. Educational Testing Service's distinguished history in computer-based testing, dating from the 1950s, has changed the face of standardized testing from the traditional multiple-choice examination.

Computer Adaptive Technologies, Inc.
Suite 2E
2609 W. Lunt Avenue
Chicago, IL 60645

Computer Adaptive Technologies offers computer-based solutions for testing and survey organizations worldwide. Product line consists of closely integrated components that address testing from applicant registration through item banking, paper and pencil test production or comput-

erized test administration and score reporting.

High Techsplanations, Inc.
Suite 902
6001 Montrose Road
Rockville, MD 20852-4874

High Techsplanations (HT) is a world leading developer of innovative virtual reality medical simulation technology. Tremendous demand exists for enhancing ways healthcare providers learn invasive procedures. HT develops systems that incorporate the visual, physical/behavioral, and tactile realism necessary for lifelike medical simulation for many prominent educational institutions and medical equipment companies.

Integrated Medical Simulation, Inc.
Suite 470N
301 4th Avenue South
Minneapolis, MN 55415

Integrated Medical Simulations, Incorporated, will demonstrate the basic tools in simulation, force feedback devices and anatomic models. Its goal is to facilitate a collaborative effort unifying the best of technology from around the world to create an affordable, useful tool for training and testing.

Knapp & Associates International, Inc.
712 Executive Drive
Princeton, NJ 08540

Computerized testing is now feasible for moderate to small certification boards, however the key to success is careful planning. Knapp & Associates International, Inc. will provide consultation and tools for planning a conversion to computerization. The exhibit will assist participants in determining the feasibility of computerization for their programs with the use of online, computerized planning tools. The critical factors necessary for a successful transition will also be identified.

National Board of Medical Examiners
3750 Market Street
Philadelphia, PA 19104

The National Board of Medical Examiners is involved in the development and implementation of computer-delivered examinations and is in the process of incorporating computer-based case simulations into licensing examinations. Computer-based testing demonstrations and information on introducing efficient testing techniques and higher fidelity simulation formats will be available.

Professional Examination Service
475 Riverside Drive
New York, NY 10115-0089

Question: What issues does a sponsor of a certification or licensure program have to address in order to move the credentialing examination from the traditional paper-and-pencil format to a computer-delivered test?
Answer: Visit the Professional Examination Service exhibit. It highlights the important points that decision-makers must think about in making the transition.

Sylvan Prometric
2601 W. 88th St.
Bloomington, MN 55431

Sylvan Prometric, a division of Sylvan Learning Systems, is the largest provider of computer-based certification and licensure examinations in the United States. The exhibit will demonstrate how multi-site standardized tests can be administered in a secure and professional environment. Secure, professional standardized test administration is available at over two hundred and twenty locations with a total of over two thousand workstations. There are Sylvan Technology Centers in every United States jurisdiction covering all major metropolitan areas.

Conference Registrants

Richard P. Anderson, MD
ABTS/Examination Sub-Cmte.
Chairman
The Virginia Mason Clinic
1100 Ninth Avenue
Seattle, WA 98101

Raymond G. Auger, MD
Neurologist/Associate Professor
Mayo Clinic
200 First Street, Southwest
Rochester, MN 55905

Robert F. Avant, MD
Deputy Executive Director
American Board of Family
   Practice
2228 Young Drive
Lexington, KY 40505

H. Randolph Bailey, MD
Examination Chairman
Univ of Texas Affil Hosp/
   Hermann Hosp
6550 Fannin St, #2307
Houston, TX 77030

Charles G. Baker, DDS
Examiner-in-Chief
Royal College of Dentists of
   Canada
365 Bloor Street, East, #1706
Toronto, ON M4W 3L4
Canada

Helena Balon, MD
Staff Physician
William Beaumont Hosp.,
   Royal Oak
3601 W 13 Mile Road
Royal Oak, MI 48073

Sorush Batmangelich, EdD
President
BATM Medical Education
   Consultants
88 Manchester Drive
Buffalo Grove, IL 60089-6767

John Becher, DO, FACOEP
Treasurer
American Osteopathic Board
   of Emergency Medicine
142 E. Ontario, #217
Chicago, IL 60611

Walter Bechtel
Assistant Director,
End User Support
University of Miami
1365 Memorial Drive
Coral Gables, FL 33146

Isaac I. Bejar, PhD
Principal Research Scientist
Educational Testing Service
Div. of Cognitive &
   Instructional Science
Mail Stop 11 R
Princeton, NJ 08541

Miriam Friedman Ben-David, PhD
Co-Director, CSA Programs
Educl Comm for Foreign
   Med Grad
3624 Market St.
Philadelphia, PA 19104

John L. Bennett, M Ed
Executive Director
American Board of
   Podiatric Surgery
1601 Dolores Street
San Francisco, CA 94110-4906

Bedford T. Bentley Jr.
Comm of Bar Admissions Admin
State Board of Law Exam
100 Community Pl., Rm. 1.210
Crownsville, MD 21032-3226

Michael A. Berry, MD, MS
Preventive & Aerospace Med
    Consultants
10777 Westheimer, Suite 935
Houston, TX 77042

Thomas W. Biester
Asst. Dir. of Evaluation
American Board of Surgery
1617 John F. Kennedy Blvd.,
    Suite 860
Philadelphia, PA 19103-1847

Eldon D. Bills, DDS
Secretary-Treasurer
American Board of Orthodontics
1421 N. Beaver St
Flagstaff, AZ 86001

David Blackmore, PhD
Director
Evaluation Bureau
The Medical Council of Canada
2283 St. Laurent Blvd
Ottawa, ON K1G 5A2
Canada

James D. Blum, PhD, CPA-IA
Director of Exams Division
A.I.C.P.A.
Harborside Financial Center
201 Plaza Three
Jersey City, NJ 07311

Andre-Philippe Boulais
Manager, Part I Examination
The Medical Council of Canada
2283 St. Laurent Blvd
Ottawa, ON K1G 5A2
Canada

L. Thompson Bowles, MD, PhD
President
National Board of
    Medical Examiners
3750 Market Street
Philadelphia, PA 19104

John R. Boyce, DVM, PhD
Executive Director
Natl Bd Examination Cmte for
    Veterinary Med
3N 081 Morningside Ave.
West Chicago, IL 60185

G. Richard Braen, MD
266 Elmwood Ave., Ste. 303
Buffalo, NY 14222

Murray E. Brandstater, MD
Loma Linda Univ Hospital
11234 Anderson St, Rm A237
Loma Linda, CA 92354

Bertha L. Bullen, PhD
Oral Exam/Research Proj. Mgr
American Board of
    Emergency Medicine
3000 Coolidge Road
East Lansing, MI 48823

Jane V. Bunce
Director of Operations
American Board of Surgery
Suite 860
1617 John F. Kennedy Blvd.
Philadelphia, PA 19103-1847

M. Desmond Burke, MD
Director, Clinical Laboratory
New York Hospital-Cornell
    Medical Center
525 East 68th Street
New York, NY 10021

Albert E. Burns, DPM
Vice-President
American Board of Podiatric
  Surgery
669 Crespi Drive, #B
Pacifica, CA 94044-3430

Michael J. Burns, DPM
American Board of Podiatric
  Surgery
1100 Poudre River Dr.
Fort Collins, CO 80524-3551

Robert W. Cantrell, MD
Executive Vice President
Dept. Otolaryngology-Head &
  Neck Surg
Univ Virginia Medical Center
Box 430 - Otolaryngology
Charlottesville, VA 22908

M. Paul Capp, MD
Executive Director
American Board of Radiology
5255 E. Williams Circle, Ste 6800
Tucson, AZ 85711

Susan S. Caulk, CRNA, MA
Director of Recertification
Council on Recertification of
  Nurse Anesthetists
222 S. Prospect Avenue
Park Ridge, IL 60068

James Cawley
Dev. Committee Member
Natl Comm on Certn of Phys Asst
214 Purlington Rd
Lutherville, MD 21093

Sally H. Chai, PhD
Director
Health Programs
American College Testing (ACT)
2255 N. Dubuque Rd
P.O. Box 168
Iowa City, IA 52243

Dane M. Chapman, MD, PhD
Program Director
York Hospital/Penn State Hershey
1001 South George St.
York, PA 17405

A. Dale Chisum, DO, FACOEP
Secretary
American Osteopathic Board
  of Emergency Medicine
142 E. Ontario, #217
Chicago, IL 60611

Gabriel Cirino-Gerena
Director
Corporacion Psicometrica
Avenue Munoz Rivera 1007
Edif. Darlington, Oficina 1203
Rio Piedras, Puerto Rico 00925

Stephen Clew
Vice Pres. of Finance, Bus. Admin.
Columbia Assessment
  Services, Inc.
3725 National Drive
Northampton Bldg, Suite 213
Raleigh, NC 27612

Nancy L. Collins, DVM
Natl Bd Examination Cmte
  for Veterinary Med
8413 Orchard St
Alta Loma, CA 91701

**Lourdes C. Corman, MD, FACP,
  FACR**
Professor & Vice-Chair
Division of Education
University of Louisville
Department of Medicine
Ambulatory Care Bldg.
Louisville, KY 40292

Della Croteau
Manager, Registration Programs
Ontario College of Pharmacists
483 Huron Street
Toronto, ON M5R 2R4
Canada

George E. Cruft, MD
Director of Evaluation
American Board of Surgery
Suite 860
1617 John F. Kennedy Blvd.
Philadelphia, PA 19103-1847

Nuria Cuevas
Director
Academic Services
NE Ohio Univ College
  of Medicine
4209 SR 44, Box 95
Rootstown, OH 44272-0095

Bruce F. Cullen, MD
Dept. of Anesthesiology,
  Box 259724
Harborview Medical Center
325 Ninth Avenue
Seattle, WA 98104-2499

Anita S. Curran, MD, MPH
Associate Dean Comm Health
UMDNJ-Robert Wood Johnson
  Med School
125 Paterson Street
New Brunswick, NJ 08901-1977

Scott Dalhouse
Administrator
American Osteopathic Assn
142 E. Ontario St
Chicago, IL 60611

Timothy J. Dalton
Managing Editor
American Board of
  Emergency Medicine
3000 Coolidge Road
East Lansing, MI 48823

Ivan Damjanov, MD, PhD
Chairman
Univ of Kansas Medical Center
  School of Medicine
Dept of Pathology &
  Laboratory Med
3901 Rainbow Blvd
Kansas City, KS 66160

Laurie Daniels
Assistant Executive Director
American Board of Obstetrics/
  Gynecology
2915 Vine Street
Dallas, TX 75204

Daniel F. Danzl, MD
4804 Smith Road
Floyd Knobs, IN 47119-9214

Jasper Daube, MD
Chair, Dept. of Neurology
Mayo Clinic
200 First Street, SW
Rochester, MN 55905

W. Dale Dauphinee, MD
Executive Director
Medical Council of Canada
2283, Bl. St. Laurent Blvd.
Suite 300
Ottawa, ON K1G 5A2
Canada

Glenn Craig Davis, MD
Vice President, Acad Aff
Henry Ford Health System
1 Henry Ford Place
Detroit, MI 48202

Lawrence W. Davis, MD
Chairman, Radiation Oncology
Emory Univ. School of Medicine
1365 Clifton Rd, NE
Atlanta, GA 30322

David R. DeMarais
Director of Testing
American Dental Assoc.
211 E. Chicago Ave.
Chicago, IL 60611

Jacques E. Des Marchais, MD
Chair, Central Exam
Medical Council of Canada
2283 Bl. St. Laurent Blvd., #300
Ottawa, ON K5G 5A2
Canada

John H. Diephouse
Exec. Mgr., Operations & HR
American Board of
    Emergency Medicine
3000 Coolidge Road
East Lansing, MI 48823

Sandra Dolan, PhD
Psychometrician
American Osteopathic Assn
142 E. Ontario St
Chicago, IL 60611

William Droegemueller, MD
UNC School of Medicine
Dept. Ob/Gyn, CB #7570
5007 Old Clinic Building
Chapel Hill, NC 27599-7570

A.J. Dunsdon
Registrar
Ontario College of Pharmacists
483 Huron St.
Toronto, ON M5R 2R4
Canada

Stewart B. Dunsker, MD
Mayfield Clinic
2123 Auburn Avenue, Suite 441
Cincinnati, OH 45219

Cynthia C. Durley, M Ed
Director
Testing & Measurement
Dental Assisting National Board
216 East Ontario Street
Chicago, IL 60611-9337

Bob Edelman
Director, Technology
Stanley H. Kaplan Educl Ctr, Ltd.
810 Seventh Avenue
New York, NY 10019

Charles Fagan
Dir of Computing Services
SIU School of Medicine
P.O. Box 19230
Springfield, IL 62794-1217

Adam S. Ferber
Director of Examinations
The State Bar of California
555 Franklin St.
San Francisco, CA 94102

Danielle Ferron
Research Associate
Royal College of Physicians and
    Surgeons of Canada
774 Promenade Echo Drive
Ottawa, ON K1S 5N8
Canada

Ben Field, DO, FACOEP
Board Member
American Osteopathic Board
    of Emergency Medicine
142 E. Ontario, #217
Chicago, IL 60611

David W. Fielding, EdD
Assoc. Professor
Pharmaceutical Sciences
University of British Columbia
2146 East Mall
Vancouver, BC V6T 1Z3
Canada

Ann Fisher
Director of Education & Info
National Conf of Bar Examiners
333 N. Michigan, #1025
Chicago, IL 60601

James Fitch
Deputy Exec. Vice President
Natl Comm on Certn of
    Phys Asst
2845 Henderson Mill Rd., N.E.
Atlanta, GA 30341

Gregory Fortna, MS, EdD
Director of Testing
Am Bd of Psychiatry
    & Neurology
500 Lake Cook Rd, #335
Deerfield, IL 60015

David F. Foster, PhD
Manager
Evaluation Services
Novell, Inc.
1555 North Technology Way
Orem, UT 84057

Howard R. Fox, DPM
Associate Professor
NY College of
    Podiatric Medicine
1800 Park Avenue
New York, NY 10035

E. John Gallagher, MD
3755 Henry Hudson
    Pkwy 14GH
Bronx, NY 10463

Alberto Galofre, MD
Associate Dean
St. Louis University
    School of Medicine
1402 S. Grand Blvd.
St. Louis, MO 63104

Bruce M. Gans, MD
Rehabilitation Inst of Michigan
261 Mack Blvd
Detroit, MI 48201

Albert B. Gerbie, MD
Chairman
American Board of Obstetrics
    & Gynecology
800 Deerfield Rd, Unit 106
Highland Park, IL 60035

Gerald S. Golden, MD
Vice President
National Board of
    Medical Examiners
3750 Market Street
Philadelphia, PA 19104

Harold E. Goodis, DDS
Director
American Board of Endodontics
1455 Jefferson St.
San Francisco, CA 94123

William E. Gotthold, MD
409 Lower Sunnyslope Rd
Wenatchee, WA 98801

Robert Greenberg
Exec. Vice President
Stanley H. Kaplan Educl Ctr, Ltd.
444 Madison Ave., #803
New York, NY 10022

Leon Gross, PhD
Dir. of Psychometrics & Research
National Board of
   Examiners in Optometry
Suite 1010
4340 East West Highway
Bethesda, MD 20814

Robert O. Guerin, PhD
Vice-President
The American Board of Pediatrics
111 Silver Cedar Court
Chapel Hill, NC 27514-1651

Dennis Guest, DO, FACOEP
Chairman
American Osteopathic Board
   of Emergency Medicine
142 E. Ontario, #217
Chicago, IL 60611

Bruce V. Gunderson, DC
President
Am Bd of Chiropractic
   Orthopedists
4211 Holladay Blvd.
Salt Lake City, UT 84124-2607

Charles L. Haine, OD, MS
Coordinator of Clin Exams
Natl Board of Examiners
   in Optometry
4340 East West Highway
Bethesda, MD 20814

Hazen Ham, PhD
American Board of
   Emergency Medicine
3000 Coolidge Road
East Lansing, MI 48823

Beth Hammond
Data Processing Manager
The American Board
   of Pathology
One Urban Centre, Suite 690
4830 West Kennedy Blvd
P.O. Box 25915
Tampa FL 33622-5915

Kerry Hamsher, PhD
Examinations Chair
Neuropsychology Clinic
University of Wisconsin
1218 W. Kilborn Ave., Ste. 415
Milwaukee, WI 53233-1325

Julie Harris
Consultant
Columbia Assessment
   Services, Inc.
3725 National Drive
Northampton Bldg, Suite 213
Raleigh, NC 27612

Aftab Hassan, PhD
Vice Pres Acad Development
Metro Academic Research
4401-A Connecticut Ave, NW,
   #291
Washington, DC 20008

Richard S. Hawe, DVM, ABVP
Natl Bd Examination Cmte for
   Veterinary Med
1210 Lyndale Dr.
Alexandria, VA 22308

John R. Hayes, MD
Medical Director
St. Vincent Hospital
2001 W. 86th Street
Indianapolis, IN 46260

Said Karim Hayez, PhD
President
Columbia Assessment Services, Inc
3725 National Drive
Northampton Bldg, Suite 213
Raleigh, NC 27612

Thomas G. Healey, CRNA
Chairman
Council on Certification
of Nurse Anesthetists
180 Leaf Street
Long Lake, MN 55356

Joseph Henkle, MD
Associate Professor
SIU School of Medicine
PO Box 19230
Springfield, IL 62794-9230

Norman R. Hertz, PhD
Manager
Office of Examination Resources
Department of Consumer Affairs
400 R Street, Ste. 1070
Sacramento, CA 95814

Kaaren I. Hoffman, PhD
Univ Southern California
School of Medicine
Research Division
1975 Zonal Ave., KAM 200
Los Angeles, CA 90033-1039

Jack Hoggatt
Office Manager
American Board of
   Podiatric Surgery
1601 Dolores St.
San Francisco, CA 94110-4906

Susan Hollister
Exam Committee Chair
Natl Certification Board for
   Therapeutic Massage
   & Bodywork
Bartlett Farm, Centerville Rd
PO Box 19
Hyde Park, VT 05655

Gerald B. Holzman, MD
Director of Education
Am Coll of Obstetricians
   & Gynecologists
409 12th Street, SW
Washington, DC 20024-2188

Barry Hornburg
Systems Analyst
American Board of Obstetrics
   & Gynecology
2915 Vine Street
Dallas, TX 75204

Victor F. Huckell, MD
Program Director
Cardiology Training
University of British Columbia
865 West 10th Avenue
West Vancouver, BC V5Z 1L7
Canada

Francis P. Hughes, PhD
Executive Secretary
American Board of
   Anesthesiology
4101 Lake Boone Trail
The Summit - Suite 510
Raleigh, NC 27607-7506

Frank B. Hurley
Director/Treasurer
Amer Bd of Cardiovascular
   Perfusion
207 North 25th Avenue
Hattiesburg, MS 39401

Harry J. Hurley, MD
Executive Director
American Board of Dermatology
39 Copley Road
Upper Darby, PA 19082

Byron L. Hutchinson, DPM
Member, Board of Directors
American Board of
    Podiatric Surgery
14212 Ambaum Blvd, SW #106
Seattle, WA 98166-1437

Lynn Johnson, PhD
Program Manager
University of Iowa
College of Dentistry
801 Newton Road
Iowa City, IA 52242

William T. Johnson, DDS, MS
Director
Am Bd of Endodontics
2503 Cae Drive
Iowa City, IA 52246

Dorthea Juul, PhD
Deputy Executive Vice President
Am Bd of Psychiatry
    & Neurology
500 Lake Cook Rd. #335
Deerfield, IL 60015

Theresa Kanya, MBA
Director, Self-Assessment
American College of Physicians
Independence Mall West
Sixth Street at Race
Philadelphia, PA 19106-1572

Amos Katz, MD
Director, Students Evaluation
Ben-Gurion Sch of Med,
    Beer-Sheva, Israel
C/O 862 B Hoover Village Dr
Indianapolis, IN 46260

Susan G. Kephart
Credentials Coordinator
American Board of
    Emergency Medicine
3000 Coolidge Road
East Lansing, MI 48823

Harry R. Kimball, MD
President
American Board of
    Internal Medicine
3624 Market Street
Philadelphia, PA 19104-2675

Larry Klein, PhD
Klein & Associates
1439 Picadilly Circle
Mount Prospect, IL 60056

Charles J. Krause, MD
Senior Assoc Dean
University of Michigan
M7300 Medical Science Bldg
1301 Catherine St.
Ann Arbor, MI 48109-0608

Becky Krumm
Development Editor
Williams & Wilkins
1400 N. Providence Rd, Ste. 5025
Media, PA 19063-2043

Deanna Williams Laws
Director of Programs
Ontario College of Pharmacists
483 Huron Street
Toronto, ON M5R 2R4
Canada

Bernard M. Lefebvre, MD
Director
Royal College of Physicians and
Surgeons of Canada
774 Promenade Echo Drive
Ottawa, ON K1S 5N8
Canada

John H. Littlefield, PhD
Dir. of Educl Research
& Development
University of Texas HSC-
San Antonio
7703 Floyd Curl Dr.
San Antonio, TX 78284

Glennis G. Lundberg
Administrative Director
American Board of Thoracic Surgery
One Rotary Center, #803
Evanston, IL 60201

John E. Madewell, MD
Chair
Department of Radiology
Penn State University
Hershey Medical Center
500 University Drive
Hershey, PA 17033

F. Patrick Maloney, MD
VA Medical Center
170 VA, Rehab Med Clinic
N. Little Rock, AR 72114

Michelle Marcy
Assistant Professor
SIU School of Medicine
PO Box 19230
Springfield, IL 62794-1217

Vincent J. Markovchick, MD
Denver General Hospital
Dept. of Emergency Med
777 Bannock St.
Denver, CO 80204-4507

Maurice J. Martin, MD
Pres, ABMS Exec Cmte
Mayo Clinic
200 First Street, SW
Rochester, MN 55905

Paul Martin
Computer Analyst
American Board of Otolaryngology
2211 Norfolk, #800
Houston, TX 77098-4044

Denise Massey
Head, Exam Production
Royal Coll Phys & Surg of Canada
774 Promenade Echo Drive
Ottawa, ON, K1S 5N8
Canada

M. Jane Matjasko, MD
Dept. of Anesthesiology
Univ of Maryland Medical System
Suite 511C
22 South Greene Street
Baltimore, MD 21201

John Mattan
Area Director
National Evaluation Systems
30 Gatehouse Road
Amherst, MA 01002

Mary Lou McGanney, PhD
Assistant Dean
New York College of
Pediatric Medicine
1800 Park Avenue
New York, NY 10035

Frederic McHale
Director, GMAT
Educational Testing Service
Rosedale Road (40-V)
Princeton, NJ 08541

Philip A. McHale, PhD
Associate Dean
Univ of Oklahoma
College of Medicine
BSMB Room 357
PO Box 26901
Oklahoma City, OK 73190

Martha Brown Menard, PhD
Member, Board of Directors
Natl Certification Board
for Therapeutic
Massage and Bodywork
250 W. Main St., #501
Charlottesville, VA 22902

John D. Milam, MD
UTHSC-H Medical School
Path & Lab Medicine
P.O. Box 20708
Houston, TX 77225

Judith Miles, MD, PhD
Professor
Univ of Missouri-Columbia
Hosp & Clinics
Dept. of Child Health
One Hospital Drive, DC058.00
Columbia, MO 65212

Robert H. Miller, MD
Chairman
Tulane Univ Med Center
Dept of Oto, Head & Neck
Surgery SL59
1430 Tulane Avenue
New Orleans, LA 70112-2699

Rodney R. Million, MD
Director, American Board of
Radiology
University of Florida
Department of Radiation Oncology
Box 100385, JHMHC
Gainesville, FL 32610-0385

Benson S. Munger, PhD
Executive Director
American Board of
Emergency Medicine
3000 Coolidge Road
East Lansing, MI 48823

James R. Neff, MD
Professor & Chairman
Orthopaedics Dept
Univ of Nebraska Medical Center
600 South 42nd St
Box 981080
Omaha, NE 68198-1080

Elizabeth Nieginski
Senior Acquisitions Editor
Williams & Wilkins
Suite 5025
1400 N. Providence Rd,
Media, PA 19063-2043

Stanley J. Niemiec, CPA
Director of Administration
Am Bd of Psychiatry
& Neurology
500 Lake Cook Rd., #335
Deerfield, IL 60015

Ronald J. Nungester, PhD
Vice-President
Client Programs & Psy.
National Board of
Medical Examiners
3750 Market Street
Philadelphia, PA 19104

Burton M. Onofrio, MD
Mayo Clinic
Department of Neurosurgery
200 First Street, SW
Rochester, MN 55905

William D. Owens, MD
Dept. of Anesthesiology
Box 8054
Washington Univ
Sch of Medicine
660 So. Euclid Avenue
St. Louis, MO 63110

Dwight K. Oxley, MD
Wesley Medical Center
Pathology Dept
550 North Hillside
Wichita, KS 67214

Louise Papineau
Head, Exam Administration
Royal Coll of Phys
    & Surgs of Canada
774 Promenade Echo Drive
Ottawa, ON K1S 5N8
Canada

Oleg Petrov, DPM
Chair, Exam Committee
St. Joseph Hospital, Chicago
111 N. Wabash Ave., #1914
Chicago, IL 60602

Thomas E. Piemme, MD
Chair
Computer Medicine Department
George Washington University
2300 K Street, NW
Washington, DC 20037

George Podgorny, MD
2115 Georgia Ave.
Winston Salem, NC 27104

Howard M. Rawnsley, MD
Trustee
American Board of Pathology
7 Haskins Road
Hanover, NH 03755

Helen C. Redman, MD
Professor
Dept. of Radiology
Univ Texas Southwestern Med Ctr
5323 Harry Hines Blvd.
Dallas, TX 75209

Mary Ann Reinhart, PhD
Deputy Executive Director
American Board of
    Emergency Medicine
3000 Coolidge Road
East Lansing, MI 48823

David S. Resch, MD
Assistant Professor
SIU School of Medicine
PO Box 19230
Springfield, IL 62794-9230

Mark G. Richmond, EdD
Executive Co-Director
Amer Bd of Cardiovascular
    Perfusion
207 North 25th Avenue
Hattiesburg, MS 39401

Wallace P. Ritchie Jr., MD, PhD
Executive Director
American Board of Surgery
Suite 860
1617 John F. Kennedy Blvd.,
Philadelphia, PA 19103-1847

Thomas J. Rohner Jr., MD
Trustee Penn State Hershey
Milton Hershey Medical Ctr
500 University Dr. C4830
Hershey, PA 17033

Rochelle Rothstein
Vice President, Health Sciences
Stanley H. Kaplan Educl Ctr, Ltd.
810 Seventh Avenue
New York, NY 10019

Raymond C. Roy, PhD, MD
Dept. of Anesthesiology
    & Perioperative Med
Med Univ of South Carolina
Rm. 525 Children's Hospital
171 Ashley Avenue
Charleston, SC 92425-2207

Judith D. Rubin, MD, MPH
Dept of Epi & Preventive
  Medicine
School of Medicine
University of Maryland
132E Howard Hall
660 West Redwood Street
Baltimore, MD 21201

William W. Ruch
President
Psychological Services, Inc.
100 West Broadway, Suite 1100
Glendale, CA 91210

Pedro Ruiz, MD
Professor & Vice Chair
University of Texas at Houston
1300 Moursund Street
Houston, TX 77030

Joseph F. Sackett, MD
Professor & Chairman
Univ of Wisconsin-Madison
  Medical School
E3/311 Clinical Sci Ctr
600 Highland Ave.
Madison, WI 53792-3252

Lawrence J. Saidman, MD
Dept. of Anesthesiology
Univ of Calif - San Diego
  Med Ctr.
9500 Gilman Drive
LaJolla, CA 92093-0815

Burton A. Sandok, MD
Consultant/Dean
Mayo Clinic
200 First St., SW
Rochester, MN 55905

Stephen C. Scheiber, MD
Executive Vice President
American Board of
  Psychiatry & Neurology
500 Lake Cook Rd., #335
Deerfield, IL 60015

Randall E. Schumacker
Family Medicine
UNT-Health Science Center
3500 Camp Bowie Blvd.
Fort Worth, TX 76107

Hugh M. Scott, MD
Executive Director
Royal Coll of Phys & Surgs of
  Canada
774 Promenade Echo Drive
Ottawa, Ontario K1S 5N8
Canada

Marie L. Shafron
Vice President for Operations
Educl Comm for Foreign Med
  Graduates
3624 Market Street
Philadelphia, PA 19104

Robert Shaw, PhD, RRT
Program Manager
Applied Management
  Professionals, Inc.
8310 Nieman Road
Lenexa, KS 66214

Linjun Shen, PhD
Director of Testing
Natl Bd of Osteopathic
  Med Examrs
2700 River Road, #407
Des Plaines, IL 60018

Paul M. Shoenfeld, DPM
Past President
Am Bd of Podiatric Orthopedics
    & Primary Podiatric Medicine
1030 S. Jefferson St, #102
Roanoke, VA 24016

Peter M. Silberfarb, MD
Chairman, Dept. of Psychiatry
Darmouth Medical School
One Medical Center Drive
Lebanon, NH 03756-0001

Ernest N. Skakun, PhD
Director of Psychometrics
Div of Studies in Medical
    Education
Univ of Alberta, Faculty of Med
2J3 Walter Mackenzie Centre
Edmonton, Alberta T6G 2R7
Canada

Joseph F. Smoley, PhD
Executive Director
Natl Bd of Osteopathic
    Med Examrs
2700 River Road, Suite 407
Des Plaines, IL 60018

Steven M. Spinner, DPM
Member, Board of Directors
American Board of
    Podiatric Surgery
301 NW 84th Avenue, #200
Plantation, FL 33324-1852

Sharon M. Stach
NABPLEX Program Director
National Assn of Boards
    of Pharmacy
700 Busse Highway
Park Ridge, IL 60068

Robert L. Stamper, MD
Chairman
California Pacific Medical Center
Dept. of Ophthalmology
2340 Clay St., 5th Fl.
San Francisco, CA 94115

James W. Stavosky, DPM
Member, Board of Directors
American Board of
    Podiatric Surgery
901 Campus Drive, #311
Daly City, CA 94015-4930

J.T. Stewart
Director, Test Development
Educl Testing Service
Georgia Office
1979 Lakeside Pkwy, #400
Tucker, GA 30084-5847

James E. Stockman III, MD
President
American Board of Pediatrics
111 Silver Cedar Court
Chapel Hill, NC 27514

Gregory E. Stone
National Certification Corp.
Suite 900
645 N. Michigan Avenue
Chicago, IL 60611

Donn A. Strand, PhD
Faculty-Med Education
Univ of Washington
3247 111th SE
Bellevue, WA 98004

Raja G. Subhiyah
Senior Psychometrician
National Board of
    Medical Examiners
3750 Market St.
Philadelphia, PA 19104

Jacques L. Surer, DO
Board Member
Memorial Hospital
1750 5th Avenue, Suite 301
York, PA 17403

James S. Tan, MD
Chairman/Program Director
Summa Health System
75 Arch Street, Suite 303
Akron, OH 44304

Peter E. Tanguay, MD
Ackerly Professor
Bingham Child Guidance Clinic
200 East Chestnut St.
Louisville, KY 40202

Paul Tannenbaum, DDS
Director
American Board of
    Periodontology
931 Fifth Avenue
New York, NY 10021

Stephen J. Thomas, MD
Dept. of Anesthesiology
New York Hospital–CUMC
525 E. 68th Street
New York, NY 10021

H. Stanley Thompson, MD
University of Iowa
Dept. of Ophthalmology
C2346H, 2000 Hawkins Dr.
Iowa City, IA 52242

James Thorne, DVM
Associate Professor
University of Missouri
College of Veterinary Medicine
100A Connaway
Columbia, MO 65211

Darwin Tichenor
Examination Specialist
Wisconsin Dept of Regulation &
    Licensing
1400 E. Washington Ave.
Madison, WI 53713

William F. Todd, DPM
Secretary-Treasurer
American Board of
    Podiatric Surgery
27483 Dequindre Road, #306
Madison Heights, MI 48071-5715

Leonard E. Toon, DC
Executive Director
Am Bd of Chiropractic
    Orthopedists
PO Box 3036
Granada Hills, CA 91394-0036

Michael J. Trepal, DPM
Member, Board of Directors
American Board of Podiatric
    Surgery
115 Henry Street
Brooklyn, NY 11201-2562

David B. Troxel, MD
Dept. Pathology
Mt. Diablo Med Ctr
2540 East St
Concord, CA 94520

Walter W. Tunnessen Jr., MD
Senior Vice President
American Board of Pediatrics
111 Silver Cedar Court
Chapel Hill, NC 27514-1651

Phil Turk
Education Systems Analyst
Society of Actuaries
475 N. Martingale, Ste 800
Schaumburg, IL 60173

Sharon Vander Weide
Education Coordinator
Bowman Gray School of Medicine
Wake Forest University
Medical Center Blvd.
Winston-Salem, NC 27157

J. Jon Veloski
Director
Medical Education Research
Jefferson Medical College
of Thomas Jefferson University
1025 Walnut St, 119 College Bldg.
Philadelphia, PA 19107

J. Whitney Wallingford
Legal Counsel, AB Family Practice
Greenebaum, Doll & McDonald
P.O. Box 1808
Lexington, KY 40593

Gerald P. Whelan, MD
820 Havana
Long Beach, CA 90804-48823

David E. Wiles, PhD
Manager, Testing Center
University of Miami
1365 Memorial Drive
Coral Gables, FL 33145

Andrew J. Wiley
Research Associate
Section for the MCAT
Assoc. of American
Medical Colleges
2450 N. Street, NW
Washington, DC 20037-1127

Caryn Wilson
Administrator
American Board of
Otolaryngology
2211 Norfolk, #800
Houston, TX 77098-4044

Barry L. Wohlgemuth, DDS
President/Project Director
Dental Interactive
Simulations Corp.
1450 S. Havana St., Suite 200
Aurora, CO 80012

Arthur Y. Wong
Director of Marketing
& Operations
Musculographics, Inc.
1840 Oak Avenue
Evanston, IL 60201

Kay H. Woodruff, MD
Brookside Hospital
Pathology Department
2000 Vale Road
San Pablo, CA 94806

James M. Woolfenden, MD
Secretary
American Board of
Nuclear Medicine
Arizona Health Science Center
Division of Nuclear Medicine
1501 N. Campbell
Tucson, AZ 85724

Paul R. Young, MD
Executive Director
American Board of
Family Practice
2228 Young Drive
Lexington, KY 40505

John W. Yunginger, MD
Executive Secretary, ABAI
Mayo Clinic
406 Guggenheim Bldg.
200 First Street, SW
Rochester, MN 44909

Committee on Study of Evaluation Procedures (COSEP)

*Elliott L. Mancall, MD
Hahnemann University–Medical
    College of Pennsylvania
Department of Neurology
Broad & Vine Streets
Philadelphia, PA 19102

George E. Cruft, MD
American Board of Surgery
Suite 860
1617 John F. Kennedy Blvd.
Philadelphia, PA 19103-1847

Joel A. DeLisa, MD
UMDNJ Medical School,
    University Heights
University Hospital, Room B-261
150 Bergen Street
Newark, NJ 07103-2406

Stewart B. Dunsker, MD
Mayfield Neurological Institute
2123 Auburn Avenue, Suite 431
Cincinnati, OH 45219

*Francis P. Hughes, PhD
American Board of Anesthesiology
4101 Lake Boone Trail
The Summit Suite 510
Raleigh, NC 27607-7506

Edward A. Krull, MD
Department of Dermatology
Henry Ford Hospital
Detroit, MI 48202

Mary Ann Reinhart, PhD
American Board of Emergency
    Medicine
3000 Coolidge Road
East Lansing, MI 48823

Fred G. Smith, MD
American Board of Pediatrics
111 Silver Cedar Court
Chapel Hill, NC 27514-1651

Conference Staff

Maxima Avila
*Philip G. Bashook, Ed.D.
Marci Burr
J. Lee Dockery, M.D.
Bobbye Higdon

Kathleen Hoinacki
Evalyn Moore
Alexis Rodgers
Gail Strejc
Kathy Szarnych

*Members Conference Planning Sub-Committee

Appendix II

Bibliography

General Topics

1. Abramson FD. A futurist view of the bar examination. *Bar Examiner*, (February) 1990: 4-17.

2. Berner ES, Webster GD, Shugerman AA, Jackson JR, Algina J, Baker AL, Ball EV, Cobbs CG, Dennis VW, Frenkel EP, Hudson LD, Mancall EL, Rackley C, Taunton OD. Performance of four computer-based diagnostic systems. *N Engl J Med*, 1994; 330: 1792-1796.

3. Branscomb AW. Common law for the electronic frontier. *Sci Am*, 1995: 160-163 (Special Issue).

4. Burdea G, Coifett P (Eds.). *Virtual Reality Technology.* New York: John Wiley & Sons, Inc.; 1994; pp. 81-116.

5. Butzin DW, Friedman CP, Brownlee RC. A pilot study of microcomputer testing in pediatrics. *Med Educ*, 1984; 18: 339-342.

6. Chidambaram L, Jones B. Impact of communication medium and computer support on group perceptions and performance: A comparison of face-to-face and dispersed meetings. *MIS Quarterly*, 1993: 465-491.

7. Greenberg DP. Computers and architecture. *Sci Am*, 1995: 120-125 (Special Issue).

8. Kapor M. Civil liberties in cyberspace. *Sci Am*, 1995: 174-178 (Special Issue).

9. Kassirer JP. A report card on computer-assisted diagnosis - The grade: C (Editorial). *N Engl J Med,* 1994; 330: 1824-1825.

10. Lee JA. The effects of past computer experience on computerized aptitude test performance. *Educ Psychol Meas,* 1986; 46: 727-733.

11. Littlewood B, Strigini L. The risks of software. *Sci Am,* 1995: 180-185 (Special Issue).

12. Lloyd JS. Computers in the future. In Lloyd, JS (Ed.): *Computer Applications in the Evaluation of Physician Competence.* Chicago, Illinois: American Board of Medical Specialties, 1984; pp. 191-193.

13. Melnick D. Computer-based testing in assessment of physician competence. *Issues,* 1988; 9: 3,7-8.

14. O'Neill KA. *Performance of examinees with disabilities on computer-based academic skills tests.* Paper presented at the Annual Meeting of the American Educational Research Association, 1995; San Francisco, CA: 1-45 (Unpublished).

15. (Panel Discussion). Problems with computers. In Lloyd JS (Ed.): *Computer Applications in the Evaluation of Physician Competence.* Chicago, Illinois: American Board of Medical Specialties, 1984; pp. 175-189.

16. Piemme TE. Computer-assisted learning and evaluation in medicine. *J Am Med Assoc,* 1988; 260: 367-372.

17. Rennie J, Press M, Rogers JT (The Editors): The computer in the 21st century. *Sci Am,* 1995: 4-9 (Special Issue).

18. Sexton-Radek K. Using computers to teach the roles of professional psychologists. *Teaching of Psychol,* 1993; 20: 248-249.

19. Sneiderman CA, Cookson JP, Hood AF. Use of computer graphic images in teaching dermatology. *Comput Med Imag Graphics,* 1992; 16: 151-152.

20. Stix G. Dr. Big Brother. *Sci Am,* 1995: 172-173 (Special Issue).

21. Studney, DR. Use of a computerized medical record for performance assessment in clinical practice. In Lloyd, JS (Ed.): *Computer Applications in the Evaluation of Physician Competence.* Chicago, Illinois: American Board of Medical Specialties, 1984; pp. 107-110.

22. Tesler LG. Networked computing in the 1990s. *Sci Am,* 1995: 10-12, 17-21 (Special Issue).

23. Vale CD. The adaptive test as a procedure for assessing competence. In Lloyd JS (Ed.): *Computer Applications in the Evaluation of Physician Competence.* Chicago, Illinois: American Board of Medical Specialties, 1984; pp. 129-134.

24. Wallich P. Tap dance. Keeping communications networks safe from bugging. *Sci Am,* 1995: 179 (Special Issue).

25. Yocom CJ. Computer-based testing: Implications for testing handicapped/disabled examinees. *Comput Nurs,* 1991; 9: 145-148.

26. Zwick R, Thayer DT, Wingersky M. Effect of Rasch calibration on ability and DIF estimation in computer-adaptive tests. *J Educ Meas,* 1995; 32: 341-363.

Computer and Adaptive Testing

27. Bergstrom BA. *Computerized adaptive testing for certification: Current issues.* Annual Meeting of the Midwestern Educational Research Association; October 1993; 1-16 (Unpublished).

28. Bergstrom BA, Stahl JA. *Assessing existing item bank depth for computer adaptive testing.* Paper presented at the Annual Meeting of the National Council on Measurement in Education; 1992; San Francisco, CA 1-14 (Unpublished).

29. Bergstrom BA, Lunz ME. Confidence in pass/fail decisions for computer adaptive and paper-and-pencil examinations. *Eval Hlth Prof,* 1992; 15: 453-464.

30. Borzo G. Professional licensing, training exams go high-tech. *Am Med News,* 1995, 38; 4.

31. Brennan RL. The conventional wisdom about group mean scores. *J Educ Meas,* 1995; 32: 385-396.

32. Buning ME, Hanzlik JR. Adaptive computer use for a person with visual impairment. *Am J Occup Ther,* 1993; 47: 998-1008.

33. Dodd BG, Koch WR, De Ayala RJ. Computerized adaptive testing using the partial credit model effects of item pool characteristics and different stopping rules. *Educ Psychol Meas,* 1993; 53: 61-77.

34. Folk VG, Green BF. Adaptive estimation when the unidimensionality assumption of IRT is violated. *Appl Psychol Meas,* 1989; 13: 373-389.

35. Green BF, Bock R; Humphreys LG; Reckase MD. Technical guidelines for assessing computerized adaptive tests. *J Educ Meas,* 1984; 21: 347-360.

36. Lunz ME, Bergstrom BA. Comparability of decisions for computer adaptive and written examinations. *J Allied Hlth*, 1991; 20: 15-23.

37. Lunz ME, Bergstrom BA. An empirical study of computerized adaptive test administration conditions. *J Educ Meas*, 1994; 31: 251-263.

38. Segall DO, Carter G. *Equating the CAT-GATB: Issues and approach.* Paper presented at the Meeting of the National Council on Measurement in Education, 1995; San Francisco, CA: 1-9.

39. Task Force, American Council on Education. *Guidelines for computerized-adaptive test development and use in education.* Washington, DC: American Council on Education; 1995.

40. Wise SL, Plake BS, Johnson PL, Roos LL. A comparison of self-adapted and computerized adaptive tests. *J Educ Meas*, 1992; 29: 329-339.

Psychometric Issues

41. Beckmann CRB, Lipscomb GH, Ling FW, Beckmann CA, Johnson H, Barton L. Computer-assisted video evaluation of surgical skills. *Obstet Gynecol*, 1995; 85: 1039-1041.

42. Bejar II. From adaptive testing to automated scoring of architectural simulations. Mancall EL, Bashook PG (Ed.): *Assessing Clinical Reasoning: the Oral Examination and Alternative Methods.* Evanston, IL; American Board of Medical Specialties, 1995; pp 115-127.

43. Bennett RE, Rock DA, Braun HI, Frye D, Spohrer JC. The relationship of expert-system scored constrained free-response items to multiple-choice and open-ended items. *Appl Psychol Meas*, 1990; 14: 151-162.

44. Bennett RE, Rock DA. Generalizability, validity, and examinee perceptions of a computer-delivered formulating-hypotheses test. *J Educ Meas*, 1995; 32: 19-36.

45. Boekkooi-Timminga E. The construction of parallel tests from IRT-based item banks. *J Educ Stat*, 1990; 15: 129-145.

46. Cass OW. Objective evaluation of competence: Technical skills in gastrointestinal endoscopy. *Endoscopy*, 1995; 27: 86-89.

47. Clauser BE, Subhiyah RG, Nungester RJ, Ripkey DR, Clyman SG. Scoring a performance-based assessment by modeling the judgments of experts. *J Educ Meas*, 1995; 32: 397-415.

48. Clauser BE, Subhiyah RG, Piemme TE, Greenberg L, Clyman SG, Ripkey D, Nungester RJ. Using clinical ratings to model score weights for a computer-based clinical-simulation examination. *Acad Med,* 1993; 68: S64-S65.

49. Diserens D, Schwartz MW, Guenin M, Taylor LA. Measuring the problem-solving ability of students and residents by microcomputer. *J Med Educ,* 1986; 61: 461-466.

50. Divgi DR. Estimating reliabilities of computerized adaptive tests. *Appl Psychol Meas,* 1989; 13: 145-149.

51. Driver R, Asoko H, Leach J, Mortimer E, Scott P. Constructing scientific knowledge in the classroom. *Educ Researcher,* 1994; 23: 5-12.

52. Ericsson KA, Charness N. Expert Performance: Its structure and acquisition. *Am Psychol,* 1994; 49: 725-747.

53. Fitzgerald JT, Wolf FM, Davis WK, Barclay ML, Bozynski ME, Chamberlain KR, Clyman SG, Shope TC, Woolliscroft JO, Zelenock GB. A preliminary study of the impact of case specificity on computer-based assessment of medical student clinical performance. *Eval Hlth Prof,* 1994; 17: 307-321.

54. Foulkes J, Bandaranayake R, Hays R, Phillips G, Rothman A, Southgate L, Wakeford R. Combining components of assessment. In Newble D, Jolly B, Wakeford R (Eds): *The Certification and Recertification of Doctors.* Great Britain, Cambridge: University Press, 1994; pp. 134-150.

55. Friedman CP, Murphy GC, Smith AC, Mattern WD. Exploratory study of an examination format for problem-based learning. *Teach Learn Med,* 1994; 6: 194-198.

56. Greaud VA, Green BF. Equivalence of conventional and computer presentation of speed tests. *Appl Psychol Meas,* 1986; 10: 23-34.

57. Kirwan JR, De Saintonge MC, Joyce CRB. Clinical judgment analysis. *Q J Med,* 1990; 281: 935-949.

58. Linn RL, Baker E, Dunbar SB. Complex, performance-based assessment: Expectations and validation criteria. *Educ Researcher,* 1991; 20: 15-21.

59. Newble D, Dauphinee D, Dawson B, Macdonald M, Mulholland H, Page G, Swanson D, Thomson A, Van der Vleuten C. Guidelines for assessing clinical competence. *Teach Learn Med,* 1994; 6: 213-220.

60. Norcini JJ. Equivalent pass/fail decisions. *J Educ Meas,* 1990; 27: 59-66.

61. Norcini JJ, Diserens D; Day SC, Cebul RD, Schwartz JS, Beck LH, Webster GD, Schnabel TG, Elstein A. The scoring and reproducibility of an essay test of clinical judgment. *Acad Med,* 1990; 65: S41-S42.

62. Norman GR. Defining competence: A methodological review. In Neufeld VR, Norman GR (Eds.): *Assessing Clinical Competence*. New York: Springer Publ Co, 1985; pp. 15-35.

63. Page EB, Petersen NS. The computer moves into essay grading: Updating the ancient test. *Phi Delta Kappan* 1995; 561-565.

64. Rothman AI; Blackmore D, Cohen R, Reznick R. The consistency and uncertainty in examiners' definitions of pass/fail performance on OSCE stations. *Eval Hlth Prof,* 1996; 19: 118-124.

65. Schnipke DL. Assessing speededness in computer-based tests using item response times. Paper presented at the Annual Meeting of the National Council on Measurement in Education, 1995; San Francisco, CA: 1-30 (Unpublished).

66. Segall DO. Equating the CAT-ASVAB: Experiences and lessons learned. Paper presented at the meeting of the National Council on Measurement in Education, 1995; San Francisco, CA: 1-11.

67. Solomon DJ, Osuch JR, Anderson K, Babel J, Gruenberg J, Kisala J, Milroy M; Stawski W. A pilot study of the relationship between experts' ratings and scores generated by the NBME's computer-based examination system. *Acad Med*, 1992; 67: 130-132.

68. Stahl JA, Lunz ME. Judge performance reports: Media and message. Paper presented at the Annual Meeting of the *American Educational Research Association*, 1991; San Francisco, CA.

69. Thompson CB, Ryan SA, Kitzman H. Expertise: The basis for expert system development. *Adv Nurs Sci*, 1990; 13: 1-10.

Security

70. Bennett CH, Brassard G, Ekert AK. Quantum cryptography. *Sci Am*, 1995: 164-171 (Special Issue).

71. Beth T. Confidential communication on the internet. *Sci Am*, 1995; 273: 88-91.

72. Eisenberg A. Privacy and data collection on the net. *Sci Am*, 1996: 274: 120.

73. Schiller JI. Secure distributed computing. *Sci Am*, 1994; 271: 72-76.

74. Stevens C. Evolution of the Internet. *Detroit News*. Detroit, MI; 95: 11A-12A.

75. Computer Security Information, World Wide Web address: http://www-ns.rutgers.edu/www-security/index.html.

Simulations Including Virtual Reality

76. Bejar II, Braun HI. On the synergy between assessment and instruction: Early lessons from computer-based simulations. *Machine-Mediated Learning,* 1994; 4: 5-25.

77. Bersky A. Computerized clinical simulation testing project (CST): Project overview and update. *Issues,* 1990; 11: 4-5.

78. Bersky AK, Yocom CJ. Computerized clinical simulation testing: Its use for competence assessment in nursing. *Nurs Hlth Care,* 1994; 15: 120-127.

79. Chopra V, Gesink J, deJong J; Bovill G; Spierdijk J; Brand R. Does training on an anaesthesia simulator lead to improvement in performance. *Br J Anes,* 1994; 73: 293-297.

80. Clyman SG, Melnick DE, Clauser BE. Computer-based case simulations. Mancall EL, Bashook PG (Eds.): *Assessing Clinical Reasoning: The Oral Examination and Alternative Methods.* Evanston, IL; American Board of Medical Specialties, 1995; pp. 139-149.

81. Devney AM. Interactive visual media for CST. *Issues,* 1990; 11: 15.

82. Dumay ACM; Jense GJ. Endoscopic surgery simulation in a virtual environment. *Comput Biol Med,* 1995; 25: 139-148.

83. Gaba DM. Improving anesthesiologists' performance by simulating reality (Editorial). *J Anes,* 1992; 76: 491-494.

84. Harless WG, Duncan RC, Zier MA, Ayers WR, Berman JR, Pohl HS. A field test of the TIME patient simulation model. *Acad Med,* 1990; 65: 327-333.

85. Henry SB, Holzemer WL. The relationship between performance on computer-based clinical simulations and two written methods of evaluation: Cognitive examination and self-evaluation of expertise. *Comp Nurs,* 1993; 11: 29-34.

86. Norcini JJ, Meskauskas JA, Langdon LO, Webster GD. An evaluation of a computer simulation in the assessment of physician competence. *Eval Hlth Prof,* 1986; 9: 286-304.

87. Saliterman SS. A computerized simulator for critical-care training: New technology for medical education. *Mayo Clin Proc*, 1990; 65: 968-978.

88. Schwartz W. Documentation of students' clinical reasoning using a computer simulation. *Am J Dis Child*, 1989; 143: 575-579.

89. Schwid HA, O'Donnell D. Anesthesiologists' management of simulated critical incidents. *Anesth*, 1992; 76: 495-501.

90. Taggert WR. Certifying pilots: Implications for medicine and for the future. Mancall EL, Bashook PG (Eds.) *Assessing Clinical Reasoning: The Oral Examination and Alternative Methods.* Evanston, IL; American Board of Medical Specialties, 1995; pp. 175-182.

91. Sidorov I. Content analysis - A personal view. *Issues*, 1990; 11: 12.

92. Swanson DB, Norcini JJ, Grosso LJ. Assessment of clinical competence: Written and computer-based simulations. *Assoc Eval Higher Educ*, 1987; 12: 220-246.

93. Tharp C. Computerized clinical simulation testing: The future is happening today. *Issues*, 1990; 11: 1, 10-11.

94. Van J. Actual side effects from virtual reality. *Chicago Tribune*. Chicago, IL; 1995: Vol. 38: 1, 3.

95. Volle RL. Standardized testing of patient management skills. *Clin Orthop Related Res*, 1990; 257: 47-51.

96. Von Schweber L, Von Schweber E. Virtually here. *PC Magazine*, 1995; 14: 168-170.

97. Webster GD. Computer simulations in assessing clinical competence: A fifteen-year perspective. In Lloyd JS (Ed.): *Computer Applications in the Evaluation of Physician Competence.* Chicago, Illinois: American Board of Medical Specialties, 1984; pp. 35-43.

98. Yam P. Surreal science: Virtual reality finds a place in the classroom. *Sci Am*, 1995: 195 (Special Issue).

Author Index

Subject Index